Praise for *So You're 70 & So You're 80*

Maralys Wills … she is clearly a force to be reckoned with.
—SIDNEY SHELDON, author of *The Other side of Midnight*

I was just going to take a peek at your book, but once started
I couldn't put it down. I love the way you write and so will
others, especially seniors. It's become my comfort book—as
some of these things were happening to me, and I didn't realize
they were happening to anyone else.
—DOROTHY NELSON, J.D.

So You're Eighty has its own distinctive lilt and balance …
science, first-hand advice, memoir, with such a lovely mix of
humor, encouragement, and inspiration … Hope people won't
wait 'til they're in their 80s to read it. You've done it again!
—STEPHANIE EDWARDS,
EMMY-WINNING MEDIA COMMENTATOR,
author of, *I Won't Be Back After These Messages*

We all learned how to parent by experience, but unfortunately
we can't learn about aging that way. Maralys' book presents a
primer on aging that is practical, humorous, and factual. I have
searched years for a resource on aging for my patients and now
I have found the perfect one. Thank you, Maralys, for helping
all of us age with dignity, grace, and humor.
—ROBIN K. DORE, M.D.

Absolutely loved it! It should be read by everyone turning 50! Maralys has a style that is down-to-earth readable. Helpful and practical in ways no one ever discusses.

—Nancy Clark,
Court-designated expert on addiction issues.

Maralys Wills' book is filled with candid, real-life examples that kept me reading—and in places laughing out loud. But more important, it contains practical information presented in an easy-to-read style—tips that will help make your good years even better.

—Irene Berardesco, B.A.

It sounds too good to be true. The title of Maralys' latest book makes me wonder: How can we really love those "Golden Years" just ahead—or already upon us? Mixing practical hints with her usual humor, Maralys gives us an enjoyable read, plus common sense strategies for dealing with the inevitable. As is her style, she draws from her own experiences, offering readers clever ways to cope.

—Linda Mayeda, M.A.

Well, Maralys, you've really done it this time. Your audience is going to relate personally to each and every chapter. Your humor is smack on.

—Jan Murra, author *Cast Off*

Fresh and funny if you're under 70. Familiar and comforting if you've been there, Maralys Wills' new book is her YouTube memories, the literary gems of her fabulous life.

—Thea Clark, PhD, author, *No! Your Other Left Foot*

So You're Eighty ... Wow!

Also by Maralys Wills

It's a Duck. And It's Dead! A Trail of Adventure
Through Six Generations

Wait for the Wind: A Romance

Revenge of the Jilted Draperies
and Other Sweet-and-Sour Stories

So You're Seventy ... So What?
How to Love the Years You Thought You'd Hate

The Tail on my Mother's Kite: A Memoir

Buy a Trumpet and Blow Your Own Horn: Turning
Books into Bucks

Damn the Rejections, Full Speed Ahead:
The Bumpy Road to Getting Published

A Clown in the Trunk: A Memoir

A Circus Without Elephants: A Memoir

Save My Son

Scatterpath: A Thriller

Higher Than Eagles: The Tragedy and Triumph of an
American Family

Fun Games for Great Parties

Soar and Surrender

A Match for Always

Mountain Spell

Tempest and Tenderness

Manbirds: Hang Gliders & Hang Gliding

So You're Eighty ... Wow!

Time to use your bag of tricks

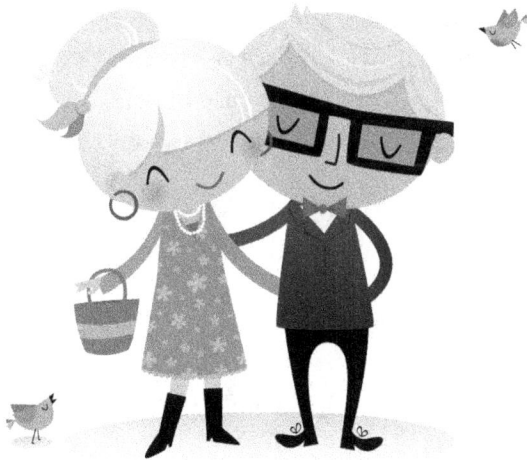

Maralys Wills

LEMON LANE PRESS • SANTA ANA, CALIFORNIA

ISBN: 978-0-578-53317-9 (print)
Also available in ebook

Book Designed by Sue Campbell Book Design

Lemon Lane Press
1811 Beverly Glen Drive
Santa Ana, CA 92705

To contact the author: maralys@cox.net
www.maralys.com

Large Print Edition

CONTENTS

Acknowledgements

No book of mine has ever been written without lots of editorial help. I'm only one mind, traveling in one limited direction—until I begin sharing what I've written with other good minds. First in line is always Rob, who's been willing, nonstop (and now for months), to put down whatever he's doing and listen to my just-written chapters. With that he comes up with chapter titles, spots misstatements or omissions, and offers better word choices. Perhaps my greatest joy as a writer is knowing Rob will be there to offer wisdom on whatever I've just created.

Next in line is my critique group—Allene, Terry, Pam, P.J., and Barbara. This second set of eyes finds the inevitable mistakes or confusing areas that eluded both Rob and me. I can't imagine trying to publish a book without their creative input.

With this volume, however, I took a new tack by calling on a wise former editor, Susan Hassebrock, to look over each chapter and suggest changes—without knowing in advance that she would also consult various authorities for additional, advisory text. Thus she has given the book important statistics that complement what was destined to be a mostly experiential approach to living through your eighties. It's my good luck—and that of my readers—that Susan was willing to address this task.

Last, but not least, a big thanks to Sue Campbell, who designed another wonderful cover and has done the large job of getting this book ready to be published. Again, I can't imagine getting into print without the important help of Sue Campbell.

A Word to the Reader

I never thought I'd write this book.

Which for me was a lot like saying, *I never thought I'd knowingly eat snails.* Clearly, some vows you stick to and some you don't.

And never mind that the snail's reputation has been prettied up with the term *escargot.* There's not enough garlic butter in the world to tempt me into consuming one of those slimy little creatures that slither across our walkways. Likewise, I never imagined I'd be writing about knee joints that creak like rusty hinges, or what brand of adult diaper doesn't leave a visible pantyline and other awkward challenges of being eighty.

But, like the garden pest I've confined to the bushes and kept off my dinner plate, the idea for this book lurked in the recesses of my mind. Little by little it crept into the light and could no longer be ignored.

Did I really want to write about this phase of life? Most of my books have been noticeably more dramatic—narratives about hang gliding, plane crashes, romance and outrageous family dramas. Was I ready to lay bare my soul and talk about things that most people avoid discussing outside of a medical office? Could I do it with compassion, dignity and the kind of humor that can only spring from personal experience?

Finally I gave in, bolstered by support and encouragement from my husband, albeit with a tiny barb.

"I can't wait to see this new book," Rob said, glancing at me over the edge of his newspaper. "You're old enough now to make some good points; you must have some wise stuff to say. Better write it down, Babe, while your memory is still working. It's gonna be great."

Well, that does it. Once more, a new book is on the way.

Still, I can't totally forget a comment by one of my writer friends: "Too bad you don't eat snails; they're so easy to catch!"

CHAPTER ONE

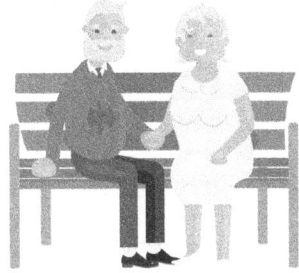

Golden Eighties:
New Challenges, New Tricks

YOU KNOW YOU'RE IN TROUBLE WHEN YOUR KIDS OR grandkids start bringing you Depends.

Bladder incontinence isn't an issue that Rob or I ever discussed with anyone, besides each other. My husband and I do have our pride, after all. Mostly we were trying to pretend that we're not quite as Senior as all those other Senior Citizens. We certainly didn't want our kids to know we were losing the embarrassing contest of mind over bladder.

However, one tiny accident in our daughter's home suddenly put Rob in that unmentionable but mortifying category. They didn't think it was funny when we explained that he was working on his ability to multi-task by laughing, sneezing and peeing at the same time. Sometimes humor is wasted on your adult kids.

As for me, my nurse/granddaughter, Lauren, did me a favor one day by bringing me a certain box. "These are pull-ups most of my patients like," she said. She slipped the box into our dressing room when I wasn't looking. For quite a while I managed to ignore the intruder as though it was left there for someone else.

"Try them, Grandma. They'll give you peace of mind," she reminded me by phone after she'd returned home. I swear I heard her mutter a muffled, "And a dry tush."

I hate to admit it, but she was right.

So there you have it. Bladders that suddenly develop minds of their own are an unmistakable sign that you just *might* be a tad more mature than you imagined.

Later that evening, after we finished watching television, I went to my computer and researched bladder control. Several sites recommended doing Kegel exercises to strengthen your pelvic floor. I didn't even know my pelvis had a floor. Okay, Kegels. I can do those. In fact, I'm already doing them, but not consistently. They're discreet, inconspicuous. No one needs to know what I'm up to. Mind over bladder, but now oftener than before.

When I did them privately that night, I whispered to Rob, "You didn't feel the bed jiggling or anything, did you?"

"Don't know what you're talking about, Babe. What was I supposed to feel?"

"Nothing," I said. "Let's get some sleep."

AFTER YOU HIT EIGHTY, YOU BEGIN NOTICING OTHER subtle changes, incidents that weren't there before. You start dozing off in places that weren't intended for napping—like theaters and lectures—while at the same time ready to pick a fight with your pillow when sleep eludes you ... such as in bed, where dreaming is supposed to come naturally.

You see yourself reflected in a storeroom window, and notice your posture has changed ... and not for the better. Quickly you straighten your shoulders. *Oh, Lord, is that old person really me?*

You become a conspiracy theorist: All kinds of dead-easy containers, like milk cartons and child-proof pill containers are suddenly, suspiciously, hard to open, inviting thoughts like, *Have they actually made this harder? Are they trying to make everything senior-proof?*

Everywhere you go, the first thing you look for is a chair. At the same time, often to your surprise, unnecessary walking sometimes makes you feel younger and better.

You purposefully head for a different room in the house, but once there begin thinking, *Okay ... What in the heck did I come for?*

Right in the middle of telling a good story, key nouns annoy you by flying out the window. "The woman's name is right on the tip of my tongue." Or, "I know it was a Baltic country, but I can't remember which one." (If you're good, like I am, at the game Taboo, which requires alternative words—you can improvise, and still make the story work.)

Handsome young men, who don't flirt anymore, hasten to hold open the door or jump up to give you their seats … because, as you eventually grasp, you are listing like a cruise ship with misaligned ballast.

IF YOU LET THEM, DISTURBING CHANGES CAN dampen what is mostly a reasonably good life. Or you can laugh them off and adjust. (*Laugh them off* is, of course, a euphemism, like *I'll run upstairs and get it.*) Neither term applies. We don't *laugh off* anything. Instead, we silently accept the unpleasant, but inevitable signs of turning eighty. Which, come to think of it, is still better than never turning eighty at all.

As to the *running upstairs for something*, each of

us has her own version. For me, it's a slow climb, one stair at a time, with a tight grip on the handrail. Which means whoever's waiting down below will simply have to wait. But usually it's my husband, Rob, who doesn't mind the delay, since he's the one who almost never climbs the stairs under any condition.

What I'm getting at is simple: at age eighty and beyond, happiness is all about two things: *attitude* and *maintenance*. But the greater of these is ATTITUDE.

As you'll see, coming up later in the book, we have a choice about Attitude ... and whether a positive outlook is just naturally in your genes, or something you've got to work at.

Meanwhile, items from our Bag of Tricks are employed every day, starting first thing each morning.

CHAPTER TWO

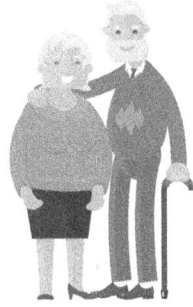

Arthritis—A Master of Disguises

I SEEM TO BE A MISTRESS OF PHONY HEART ATTACKS.

The first time, probably about my late 60s, I awoke abruptly with pains across my upper chest. *Oh, Lord, I'm having a heart attack,* I thought, but since I wasn't quite sure—not sure enough, anyway, to roust Rob out of bed—I hopped in the car and drove myself to the emergency room.

The hospital took me seriously; they performed a few tests, proved to everyone's satisfaction that those rapidly-disappearing jabs had nothing to do with my heart, brought in a tray of breakfast, and handed me papers which basically said, *you're free to leave.*

I arrived home before Rob even woke up. The difference in our day being, that I was fed and he wasn't.

I ADMIT IT ... I'VE LONG BEEN SO WELL-ACQUAINTED with my body that I notice every little thing that seems *different*, whether it's important or not. And doubtless so do others—especially those on the verge of being a hypochondriac, which it seems I am.

Trouble is, for years I've read too much but known too little.

Nevertheless, I twice saved my own life by taking a Miss Marple approach to tracking down odd symptoms, which eventually led to early stage cancers. One was breast, the other colon. Luckily, both were caught in plenty of time.

IN RETROSPECT, THOSE PAINS THAT SENT ME TO THE hospital for my first "heart attack" could have been arthritis.

If I were to guess which health issues are likely to plague an 80-year-old who's free of life-threatening diseases, most people would say arthritis.

It's an ailment that doesn't kill us, but instead begins hitchhiking on our ligaments, tendons, and joints before most of us feel we're anything close to "old."

All by itself, arthritis attacks our spines, and gravity narrows the spaces between discs and makes us shorter. Meanwhile, arthritis plays havoc with knees and hips, creating enough pain so we flock to orthopedic surgeons, demanding relief.

What many of us end up with (including both Rob and me), are replacement joints, which happily seem to make an important difference—at least in *those* joints.

How great it would be if we, the afflicted, could throw a switch and say, *Okay, you've had your fun. Now STOP.*

It doesn't work that way.

The disease marches on, twisting fingers (sadly not

replaceable), and causing a variety of peculiar pains, which, though fleeting, can briefly masquerade as something serious.

Thus one morning at three a.m., it happened again. While on a family vacation in Northern California, (now in my 80s), I woke my granddaughter Lauren, the nurse, and said "I can't be sure of this, Lauren, but I think I'm having a heart attack." I explained that the pains radiating across my chest were bad enough so they'd actually roused me from a deep sleep.

Lauren said, "Okay, Grandma, throw on your clothes. Let's go," and she promptly drove me to the nearest hospital.

As a first step, the emergency physician ordered an aspirin, then did an EKG. By now I was feeling embarrassed, even chagrined, because like that earlier time, the pains had subsided. Still, the visit included an MRI, and a variety of other tests.

My orthopedic surgeon son, Chris, staying with a nearby relative, drove on home without stopping at the hospital. I was annoyed that he'd been so cavalier about my condition. But hey, I don't hold grudges. And anyway, as I learned later, he'd made a call to the attending doctor, who reassured him that I was not in any danger.

Ever since, I've been the subject of family razzing about my "fake" heart attack … the one they know about, that is. But how was I to grasp that this was an example of arthritis masquerading as something else? Besides, we gals have long been advised, from every-where, that dangerous heart symptoms in women are markedly different from those suffered by men.

For us, problems with our hearts can pretend to be a sore shoulder, an aching jaw, fleeting pains the width of our chests, a sharp pain in the back. Even an upset stomach.

But four out of five of those symptoms can also be a harmless first cousin … arthritis.

Lately I've noticed, to my annoyance, that gnawing pains across your tailbone area can radiate into your stomach, making you feel uncomfortably full, even slightly nauseous. The hypochondriac side of my brain imagines cancer, but my more reasonable self knows it's probably just my old friend, arthritis.

Doctors suggest over-the-counter meds, moderate exercise, and the application of heat or ice—whichever works. One website recommends "gentle massage of the affected area." *Rob? I could use a little help here.*

"Glad to," he says. In all honesty, I know what he's thinking. *Anything to get my hands on her bottom.*

HOW DO WE EIGHTY-YEAR-OLDS GO ON LIVING WITH this mean-spirited culprit? How do we keep to a minimum its intrusion into our lives?

For some, our doctors will suggest an over-the-counter analgesic like Excedrin or Tyenol. Or alternatively, an OTC anti-inflammatory such as aspirin, Advil, Alleve, or Motrin. For others, a prescription might include one or more daily doses of Voltarin or Celebrex.

Each patient is different, and obviously not all medications work the same in all people. In fact, over the years I've had long stretches with a variety of different prescriptions. As individual patients, WE don't react the same way, either, to pharmaceuticals that worked just fine yesterday but are basically useless today.

Several times a year, when the arthritis pains gang up on me, jumping from one site to another and sometimes all at once, I go to my rheumatologist for a shot of a Cortisone compound (Depo-medrol), which seems to calm things down. However, I'm warned that this remedy is limited to only periodic injections per year.

The medicinal approach is always something you work out with your own doctor—hopefully someone who's known you and your body's inclinations for years.

Meanwhile, what can we do, beyond the doctor's input, to make our lives better? Come to think of it, how deep must we dig into our "bag of tricks?"

For me, and doubtless others, one of the answers is *sleep*. After an extra hour of deep sleep—meaning eight and a half hours instead of seven and a half, I'm apt to feel pretty good all day. My Tylenol, slow-acting in my case, reacts just fast enough so I'm mostly free of pain until bedtime.

Just feeling NORMAL, as though my body has backed up to age forty, becomes a kind of *high*, practically a cause for celebration.

Yet thanks to our cranky bladders, aching joints, and other gratuitous wake-up calls, a good sleep for seniors is as elusive as a wet bar of soap—one minute you've got it and the next it's shooting out of your grasp and skittering across the shower floor.

How we envy our grandkids who seem able to drop off at a moment's notice and wake up eight or nine hours later.

In fact one of my grandsons recently confided that he sometimes sneaks off from his job, finds a cot, and drops into deep sleep for something under half an hour. "Afterwards," he says, "I feel as good as if I'd just slept a whole night."

He may be on to something. A study by the

National Sleep Foundation says short naps can improve mood, alertness and performance. My napping grandson is in renowned company: Winston Churchill, John F. Kennedy, Ronald Reagan, Albert Einstein, and Thomas Edison were all known to enjoy an afternoon snooze.

A later chapter will cover both the importance of sleep to general health and well-being, and how to get more of it.

As you'll discover in the next chapter, certain pills and a good night's sleep aren't the only remedies for arthritis.

CHAPTER THREE

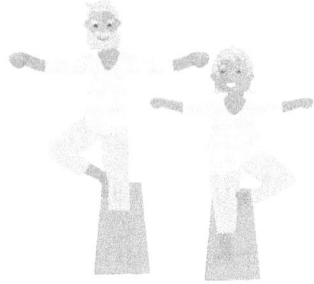

A Multi-Pronged Counter Attack

I WAS ONCE FIVE FEET TEN AND A HALF.

Unlike those awkward grammar school days when I was the tallest girl in the class with the biggest feet (and disliked looming over the boys), I graduated from UCLA at five-ten and reveled in being tall. Then, inexplicably after having several kids I found I'd grown another half inch. How nice was that! Tall was great in many ways—for tennis and clothes and high kitchen cupboards.

Now, thanks to gravity and the march of time, the

discs in my back have narrowed, and I'm only five-foot-seven. "You've shrunk!" exclaim my younger friends. "I remember having to look way up when we talked!" They don't mind the change ... but I do.

Well, that's aging for you. Along with arthritis. But with the right tricks you can live with it ... and yes, still be happy.

OSTEOARTHRITIS, THE MOST COMMON OF THE VARious types, affects 27 million Americans. Among the 65 and older crowd, almost 50 percent report doctor-diagnosed arthritis, according to statistics from the Center for Disease Control. According to my orthopedic-surgeon son, Chris, in our age group, the percentage is closer to 100%.

IF THERE'S ANY MAGIC TO BE FOUND AGAINST THE onslaught of years, one key might be exercise. Almost everyone agrees, but research physicians are adamant.

Most people assume arthritis is an inevitable part of aging, but the American Academy of Orthopaedic

Surgeons, in its publication, OrthoInfo, says it is due more to disuse than aging. Fewer than 10 percent of Americans exercise regularly and people over 50 are the most sedentary.

A documentary of 85-year-old Ruth Bader Ginsberg shows her working out with weights and doing floor routines that would be challenging for a woman in her 40s. I was astounded when I saw her doing The Plank.

Many years ago I was briefly a jogger, and I also played a lot of tennis. The first I merely endured, but the second I loved.

Early in my running days I discovered that endless cycles around a track were agonizing, partly because my legs were in open rebellion, and ultimately because the entire effort was so boring. Immediately after I finished, a slow mile or even two, I experienced a mild version of "runner's high." But later I was apt to feel sick—which was scary.

Back then, in my 40s, a doctor performing a physical had viewed certain x-rays and proclaimed, "You have a sixty-year-old back." However, since I had no symptoms, I passed off his concerns. (By now my back must be about 120.)

The running drew to a fast close. But not the tennis. From age 30 to my early 70s, I reveled in the sport; here was exercise which involved friendships, strategy, teamwork, and points. Those quick, sideways dashes were fun, especially when you reached the ball in time.

And then one day after a layoff, I was out on the court lurching for a drop shot. I was horrified when my upper body moved but my feet didn't, and I collapsed in a heap. What a jarring revelation, realizing that various parts of me were no longer synchronized.

To my dismay, my body had called a halt to tennis, but I soon found other ways to exercise. Years earlier, Rob had brought home a book titled, *Be A Loser*, by Greer Childers, which promised that a certain set of exercises would produce a significant loss of weight. Like others my age, I was perpetually on the prowl for ways to be thinner.

Following the book, page by page until the exercises became second-nature, meant only minor benefits in the weight department ... but I would eventually grasp their importance in fighting the back pains of arthritis.

Those yoga-like moves involved some funny faces and a lot of on-the-floor stretching, which my grandkids found hilarious—especially the comical faces. When I started, most were still under 10, and we have pictures of them with their tongues hanging out, imitating the weird-face parts of the routine.

Because they take only about 10 minutes I've hardly missed a day, doing my routine faithfully for years ... which I now refer to as my "Huff and Puffs."

ONE BUSY DAY WHEN I DIDN'T HAVE TIME TO DO them at home, I decided I could accomplish the face part while at the hair dresser's, waiting for the color to "take." To avoid making a scene, I snuck into a corner and began the tongue-out portion of my "workout."

I wasn't as inconspicuous as I thought. A much

too perky receptionist zipped around the corner and froze in alarm when she saw my contorted features.

"Shall I call an ambulance?" she asked. Apparently she thought I was having a seizure.

That was the last time I ever tried doing my Huff and Puffs in public.

EVENTUALLY CHRIS REMARKED THAT THOSE EXERcises had to be the reason my back wasn't giving me fits. He asked the name of the book so he could relay it to his patients. If I, with my terrible-looking X-rays, was still pain free (at least in that area), there must be a lot of value in pure, energetic stretching.

Later, because my now-grown grandkids were so impressed, I added a strenuous element called The Plank, which involves suspending your body between upper-arms and toes—in my case for a count of fifty. It was a revelation to see RBG doing them as well.

I revel in comments from my now-adult grandkids: "Look what grandma is doing!" Those Huff and Puffs aren't my only form of exercise—but that will be covered in another chapter.

ALL OF US HAVE HEARD A CERTAIN MANTRA ABOUT exercise: *No pain, no gain.* As a determined German, I once believed this dictum, and "carried on," adding pain to muscles that already hurt. Eventually those parts rebelled and refused to work at all.

This is an oft-mentioned scenario, gathered from friends who recover from surgery by going for physical therapy. A few therapists operate on the theory, "If a little exercise is good, a lot must be better." Recently, a friend said, "The therapist was so pushy he ruined my new knee, which was practically healed. He set me back weeks."

Wiser now, I operate on a different theory: *Never hurt the hurt.* Pain is nature's way of warning us. When some part of me rebels, I give it a few days' rest. Quite soon, the affected area thanks me by returning to full function.

SO NOW, WITH THREE WELL-ACCEPTED MEANS OF attacking arthritis, there remains a fourth remedy … a tactic I've read about but haven't yet tried—namely, seeing what happens when you "go off sugar."

Here and there I've read that sugar is a major cause of human inflammation … and what is arthritis, really, except inflammation on steroids?

So far, my only sessions of sugar-avoidance have been tied to high doses of Vitamin C when it's obvious I'm about to catch a cold. Unlike Rob, I'm a dedicated believer that you can ward off illness (most of the time), by starting your regimen at the first symptom—with massive doses of C and total avoidance of sugar. Sweets, I've discovered, can undo the palliative effects of the Vitamin C.

Sticking to this routine means I'm almost never sick. In fact, I've got a good friend, a Federal appellate court judge, who is such a believer in this remedy that now, at nearly 90, she says, "Thanks to my trust in Vitamin C, I've never been sick for more than one day in my entire life."

Based on these observations, I have to wonder: How does sugar-avoidance work with arthritis?

At the moment I simply I don't know.

The trouble with fully testing thus hypothesis is that I'm something of a sugarholic. Though my weight is now under control, thanks to a modicum of restraint, I can't refuse at least one scoop of ice cream or a couple pieces of See's Candy. How dull life would be if you couldn't look forward to the occasional treat.

For both Rob and me, dinner is never quite complete without dessert. Yet both of us are concerned with tamping down arthritis. If sugar really is the enemy, our joints might be healthier on a diet free of the stuff, but I'm afraid our moods would take a turn for the worse.

Until someone can prove to me that this method "works," I'll follow the old adage about keeping your friends close and your enemies closer: The See's is not going anywhere.

SO FAR, AS THE NEXT CHAPTER WILL PROVE, MY "BAG of tricks" is far from depleted.

CHAPTER FOUR

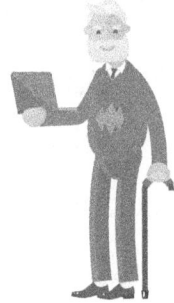

Numb Fingers: Giving Them Some Help

WHILE ROB AND I HAVE LEARNED TO COPE WITH THE various inconveniences of growing older (you notice I don't use the term *old*), we resort to ever more colorful curses and sometimes, even, to laughter.

Among those vexing tribulations Rob and I have both experienced involve fingers which have abruptly turned numb. That may sound like a mere nuisance, but when you can't feel your fingers it's hard to pluck small scraps of paper off the floor ... or small anything off of anywhere.

Even worse is trying to poke a button through a slot in your blouse when some of your digits have no sensation. Operating the tiny lobster clasp on your necklace becomes nearly impossible. For that matter, it's a challenge to force numb fingers to behave any- where. How innocently I duck the now-impossible job of shuffling cards.

These issues may seem insignificant, but they can become an ever growing sense of frustration. Think how stressful it is to always be running late because you've spent an extra fifteen minutes trying to fasten your jewelry.

As my own, *ever-on-duty* doctor, I've attributed numb fingers (Peripheral Neuropathy in medical terms), to the start of using a cane, which involved unaccustomed pressure on my right palm. With that I began backing off, caning my way only during longish walks ... or on routine strolls up and down our cul-de-sac.

While I hope, naively, that the fingers will suddenly

thank me by reverting to normal sensation, at least they've grown no worse.

Rob is also convinced that the neuropathy in his right hand is due to his several years of cane use, especially considering the additional weight he puts on the handle. As evidence, he submits his left hand, which he notes is mostly without numbness.

Further proof that the cane is the guilty party are the sharp, almost electrical shocks he often experiences in three of his fingers when using the offending prop. Yet he knows he must rely on it because his latent dizziness puts him at risk for falling.

NATURALLY OUR ORTHOPEDIC SURGEON SON, CHRIS, has an answer. "It's not your fingers, Mom, it's a deterioration of the nerves in your neck. Try doing these neck exercises," and he gave me a single sheet, complete with drawings that show the various stretching routines we numb-handers are supposed to follow. Besides suggested repetitions for each item, we're told they should be performed daily with warm, damp compresses to the neck.

A few calculations suggested that, done right, these new exercises might tack on at least fifteen extra minutes to our everyday chores—not much, of course, until they're added to everything *else* we're doing.

Besides, my rheumatologist came up with a different answer. "See this finger?" she asked, pointing to my long and crooked middle finger. "It's bent, so the nerve is incapacitated right here, where the tip goes off to one side."

"Oh," I said. And with that, the German in me set about fixing whichever root cause proved to be right.

For starters, because I'm already committed to so many health-related routines, I've resorted to shortcuts.

During the end of a daily shower, it's easy to spend a few extra minutes stretching your neck—with the hot water already beating down nicely on the affected part. I'm thinking, *Isn't this as good as a warm compress?*

If it isn't, the choice is between a surplus of tedious

exercises and getting on with *living.* There isn't time for both.

At the very least, the neck exercises make it easier to turn my head in either direction.

Still, in case the rheumatologist is right, I find myself physically bending that crooked finger into a straightened position. Which probably won't help, but it's worth a try, and besides, it's something you can do while you're listening to music at the philharmonic.

Unlike the easily-spotted tongue-out routine, nobody notices what you do with your hands … meaning nobody suggests calling an ambulance.

STILL, THE NUMB FINGERS JOURNEY MAY NOT BE finished: Months after the above was written, Chris suggested another remedy. "Mom, you might want to get a shot of Cortisone in that right wrist."

"Won't it hurt?" I asked.

"Not at all. You'll hardly feel it." He suggested I visit his former partner, another orthopedic surgeon.

And indeed, Chris' partner suggested that many

cases of numb fingers are caused by what is called Carpal Tunnel Syndrome. After a definitive test, the surgeon said that I was a candidate, and that a shot of Cortisone in the affected wrist could reduce tension on the Carpal ligament. Long term treatment would involve Carpal Tunnel Surgery, which is apparently common.

As Chris promised, the shot was painless. Time will tell whether, or how much, the shot will help—and whether surgery will be a final answer.

MEANWHILE, SOMETIMES AT NIGHT MY HANDS revolt and begin to throb. For that, my rheumatologist suggested arthritis gloves. They practically eliminate the pain and are easily purchased at a medical appliances store, or on Amazon. But they come in only one color—black—which seems a little dramatic for bedtime attire. The first night I wore them, Rob said, "Here we are, and you're going to bed with black hands, like a cat burglar."

When numb fingers continue to be a problem, it's time for tricks—namely, magnets, Velcro, and small tools.

Over the years a friendly jeweler has been converting my cranky jewelry clasps into magnets, which require zero effort, meaning you can pop them on as you go out the door. And all but my tennis shoes are now fastened with Velcro.

For shirts that button in back, I'm lucky to have a willing husband. Still, I've considered taking a few such items to our local alterations shop, Make It Fit, asking if they can substitute Velcro closings for buttons. How easy it would be to get dressed if all our clothes were fastened with velcro.

Meanwhile, back in the kitchen, Rob and I currently use a variety of numb-finger gadgets. We have grippers that help us open stubborn jar lids. For certain "convenient" tin cans with a tab opener (which, for us, aren't convenient at all), we've found a small *whatsit* called a tab-lifter that leans into the top of the lid and provides needed leverage. Other jobs require pliers ... and new and colorful curse words.

On a daily basis we receive catalogs that prove a lot of innovators have found a senior market for their gadgets.

As explained in chapter two, certain stretching exercises work especially well for arthritic spines. On the other hand, we've all been told repeatedly that even as seniors we're likely to live longer and healthier lives if we make aerobic exercise a daily part of our lives.

Among the suggestions are such simple ploys as parking one's car blocks away from stores and walking the added distance. Or finding excuses within your home to jump up and fetch distant objects.

In our neighborhood we see numerous couples out for early morning or late-afternoon strolls—with or without their canine pets.

Among my friends, quite a few go to their local gyms to participate in organized group routines. My daughter, Tracy, with friends and family, often rides her electric bike 20 or more miles down dedicated bike paths to the beach. Chris and wife Betty-Jo take regular, two-mile walks in and around the neighborhood.

Until driven indoors by summer heat, I did a 20-minute stint round and round our cul-de-sac. I can't say I ever relished walking for its own sake—I only enjoyed "having done it."

Later I resumed riding my stationery bike—and here was exercise you could love. I don't have to deal with the weather, worry about stepping in potholes, or being confronted by the occasional coyote. And best of all, while my legs carry on by themselves, I can hold a newspaper or book and read, free of that nagging voice telling me I should be doing something "productive."

Not so long ago I also read while I walked on the treadmill, which required a hanging book stand and a magazine with extra-large print.

When it comes to physical activity, my husband

and I are not exactly on equal footing. Though Rob at 92 uses a cane full time, he is still able to walk more rapidly than I do toward such places as the theater. Mother Nature probably credits him for all his years of strenuous workouts at the gym and now allows him to do more than his share of sitting.

Despite the pep in his step when we're out on the town, we both know he needs to use our treadmill at home on a more consistent basis. Even with his severe arthritis, if I issue gentle "reminders" at the right time, he'll give it a good ten to 15 minutes.

Rob shares my enthusiasm, both for staying active and for penning this book. In fact, when I escape from the kitchen to write, he's apt to support me by taking over some of my chores, even the nuisance jobs, such as cleaning the orange juicer. At our ages we both need all the encouragement we can get.

And now, with his advice, I'm about to start a chapter about some additional hassles ... the perils of using a cane.

CHAPTER FIVE

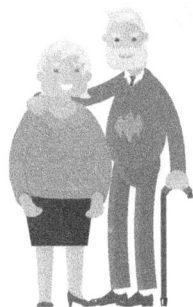

Your Extra Leg—A Cane

TEENAGERS HAVE TO PASS A DRIVING EXAM BEFORE their parents hand over the keys to the family sedan. Perhaps "old-agers" should take a test before they operate their first walking cane.

Canes are wonderfully useful, providing added stability as you walk, like having a friend to lean on. But if handled haphazardly, they can literally take the user for an unexpected spin.

Rob takes his almost everywhere. But beware! Like a puckish trickster, a cane can turn on you in an instant, smiling one minute and gleefully dumping you over the next.

Nobody knows this better than Rob and me who, between us, have taken three different spills. Each time the cane was the centerpiece of the fall—yet the fault, we had to admit, was all ours ... and only because we hadn't fully grasped the potential for a cane-induced mishap.

How well I remember where and how I happened to hit the floor. I was propelling myself along in our local CVS drugstore, heading for the pharmacy. As I rounded a corner to my right, moving quickly from one aisle to another, I swung the cane out ahead of me—and there it was, right in my own path. Before I realized I was in trouble, my foot caught the obstacle and I plunged to the ground, landing right on my face.

Thank heavens the floor was carpeted. For a moment I stayed where I was, lying on my side, not sure whether or not I was seriously injured. I felt my cheek. No blood. But I wasn't ready to do more than try to sit up.

Of course people came running. And of course I was mortified that I'd created a scene. As between a bruised cheek and embarrassment, the latter felt worse. Someone asked, "Are you all right? Shall we call an ambulance?" (After a certain age, you have to get used to people assuming you need an ambulance.) "I think I'm okay," I said, once more feeling my face. "Let me just sit here a minute." A pause. "I think it was the cane. I must have fallen over it." I wanted to say, "It jumped right in front of me," but was afraid bystanders would question my sanity as well as my physical condition.

Eventually a strong man pulled me to my feet, and I knew the damage was minimal—just a scraped cheek and nothing more. As an additional, gallant gesture, he extended his arm, let me slip mine through his, and walked me to my car.

That fall may have prevented some future, worse injury, because I'm now alert to the possibility that a cane is not always your friend, especially when a change of directions puts the thing in your path. Now, if I'm out walking and ready to turn left or right, I make sure the cane is swung wide, out of my own way.

Rob, too, ever the experienced "caner," once took a spill over his own implement. One day he was in our family room, making a right turn around a table when the cane presented itself as a sudden obstacle to his progress. He fell over it. Hard. For long moments he lay on the rug, unable to rise. I was horrified.

Not strong enough to get him to his feet, I called our nearby granddaughter, Kelly, and she and husband Matt came running. Together, the two hoisted Rob under his arms and into a chair. We were grateful that they presented such a strong and unified team.

After one spill apiece, we are both alert to the hazards of making a turn which places the cane right where you intend to walk.

EVEN MORE DANGEROUS IS THE CANE WHICH HITS A patch of wet floor or pavement. Nothing is more slippery than a rubber tip skidding across a wet surface. Unfortunately, I wasn't home when Rob took his second fall after his cane encountered a small puddle left by a melting ice cube.

As he later described his out-of-control spill, I cringed. Trouble was, his entire weight bore down on the stick—which suddenly had no "purchase," as the expression goes.

It took him considerable time to inch his way over to the family room couch, where he was able to grab a leather arm and hoist himself to his feet.

Rob's mini-disaster reminded me of children who take impressive falls as they dash across the wet area that surrounds a swimming pool. All of us have heard an adult admonishing a small child, "Walk, Sally! Don't run near the pool. It's dangerous."

The same principle applies to seniors who forget about the skid-potential of a cane on wet pavement. For a child such a fall might mean a temporary bruise.

For many a senior, the consequences can be deadly. Statistics from the University of California, San Francisco, indicate almost five million Americans use a cane of some sort. There's a host of reasons why seniors choose to use such an implement. Weak muscles, arthritis-stiffened joints and balance issues due to inner ear problems are among the likely problems.

When you're in your twenties, you can scale a mountain without a hint of vertigo, but after you hit your eighties, the slightest hitch can throw you off balance. But if you refuse to give up and take the rest of your life sitting down, you'll have to rely on that third leg.

CANES CAN BE SUMMARIZED IN ONE PHRASE: YOU love 'em, you hate 'em, you lose 'em. Oh, yes, among their annoying humanoid traits, canes have a way of hiding—in market baskets, behind a door, or deep in your car. To avoid their becoming someone else's property, we've labeled ours with return-address stickers. For those concealed within the house, finding them again is like reuniting with a lost child— you're both mad at the thing, but overjoyed to see it once more.

And here I have a story about a once-student. She and a friend were on a recent cruise and were enjoying Bloody Marys and the view from the poolside bar when one of them looked down at the cane she used for her "bad" knee. She turned and exclaimed to her friend, "This is not my cane. I've never seen this one before in my life." They never figured out where the imposter came from or what had happened to hers.

AND SPEAKING OF SLIPPERY SURFACES, AND OTHER ways you can slide …

CHAPTER SIX

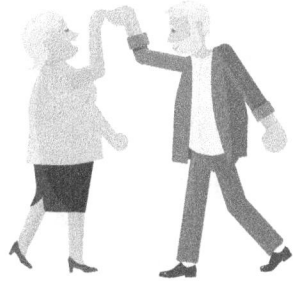

No Tubs, Safe Showers

WHEN YOU ARE YOUNG, DOING SOMETHING DANGER-
ous might mean driving too fast on the German auto-
bahn, skiing into avalanche territory, bull running
in Spain, or bull riding in Texas (well, pretty much
anything involving bulls), but for the over-eighty
crowd, navigating a slippery bathroom can be just
as hazardous.

Similar to plopping your walking cane into a puddle, trying to move bare feet across the wet surface
of a tub or shower can be equally risky. A study by

the National Institute on Aging estimates that more than one third of seniors over age 65 slip and fall each year, and 80 percent of those mishaps occur in the bathroom. Further statistics from the Centers for Disease Control and Prevention say that seniors who fall and break a hip have a 25 percent chance of dying within six months to a year after the incident. However, it's usually not the break itself that is at fault, but more often the patient's long period of inactivity.

But there are ways that you can minimize your risk.

Rob and I have stayed in some fancy (but ancient), European hotels whose only shower was contained in a deep bathtub. Tub bathing has gone out of fashion with most Californians who, like Rob and me, prefer a well-appointed walk-in shower. Besides, expecting an 80-year-old to lift her leg and ascend the steep side of a bathtub is like asking her to climb over a two-foot wall.

Even worse is when it's a tub enclosure without handholds. It took my nurse grand-daughter, Lauren, to explain how such a chore could be accomplished.

"First you sit on the side of the tub," she said. "Then, while balanced, you hoist one leg over the edge. Then the other. From there it's safe to stand up. That is, if you have hand-holds or a non-slip surface." She grinned. "You reverse the whole process getting out."

The last time we traveled with Lauren and Dan, a year ago, we gave them the regal suite in our York hotel because it sported only a tub shower ... while Rob and I took the room-with-limited-view so we could use its walk-in facility. For us a great view was not worth the hassle required of bathing in that swimming pool of a tub.

SPEAKING OF TUBS AND SHOWERS: THOUGH ROB AND I have a generous sunken shower with hand-holds all around, he discovered one day it was dangerous for him—with his soft, glassy-soled feet—to try and move across the shower's smooth tile surface. Even with those handholds, he found himself skidding. So the day after he slid into the lower water spout and slashed his knee, I went out and bought a non-slip rubber mat. Even then I needed help from the sales lady.

"This one gets slippery," she said, pointing, "when it's covered with soap. This other one remains non-slip under all circumstances." And indeed, its surface felt nubby, and impervious to water and soapy bubbles and soft feet.

So far, with the new mat, Rob feels secure in our shower. Though until he turned 91, our facility seemed perfectly okay.

OUR ISSUES CONTINUE—YET WE KEEP FINDING NEW ways to adjust.

CHAPTER SEVEN

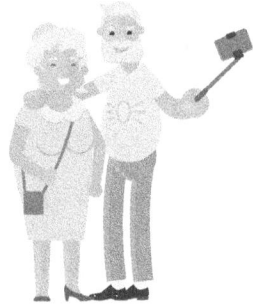

The Eyes Have It

As curious kids, I can remember that sometimes we asked each other, *Which do you think would be worse, losing your eyes or your ears?* Since none of us had cell phones back then, or even television, we had plenty of time to ponder such serious but unanswerable questions.

In fact, I even remember wondering aloud where babies came from—and this in spite of the fact that for a few years I lived on a farm where, to my brother's and my juvenile amusement, bulls regularly jumped on the backs of cows.

We kids tried to imagine a life where you couldn't see where you were going, or couldn't hear the people who spoke to you. But since none of my acquaintances back then were so afflicted, the topic was soon dropped for lack of interest.

Now, at an age where both sight and sound can be in jeopardy, I'm acutely aware that Rob and I, and most of our fellow seniors, are intent on retaining all the sight and hearing we can. To give up either would be a huge loss, possibly depriving us of the independence, mobility, and social interactions that enhance the quality of our lives.

AGE FIFTY SEEMS TO BE A TURNING POINT FOR THE accuracy of our eyesight. About then avid readers begin noticing that the print in newspapers and books seems to be getting progressively smaller, making the words difficult to discern without reading glasses. Presbyopia, as this condition is called, is a normal part of aging and may continue to worsen with time. Cartoons are apt to depict seniors holding their newspapers ever farther away. But longer arms don't seem to solve the problem.

At first simple magnification (a.k.a. "readers" from the drugstore), solves the problem. But eventually, especially for those with astigmatism, patients flock to their ophthalmologists for testing and a prescription for glasses.

A recent edition of the *Los Angeles Times* featured a well-researched article on the inherent greed behind what is often an outrageous price for prescription glasses. The trouble began with one company's monopoly on frames, which probably involve no more than ten dollars to produce, but can cost consumers two to five hundred dollars. It seems that Luxottica (perfect name for a company that turns a necessity into a luxury), has licensed numerous other outlets to carry its frames, all at the same inflated prices.

Adding prescription lenses to such frames can be another startling expense ... an arrangement that few providers wish to curtail.

I was surprised that the author never mentioned the one provider of glasses and frames that I know personally to be reasonable ... namely, Costco.

For years—probably when the price of eyewear began soaring into the stratosphere—Rob and I have replaced broken glasses or secured new ones from that same national discount store. As an added attraction, mine are fitted with transition lenses, meaning they turn into dark glasses when I'm outside in the sun. Thus I never have to bother carrying (and perhaps losing), an extra pair of dark glasses.

Recently Rob and I were at a concert listening to Itzhak Perlman as he played his violin accompanied by a 13-member orchestra. Born in 1945, he is now 73 and, as expected, wears glasses. Out of curiosity, I studied his colleague's faces to see how many also wore spectacles, and arrived at eight out of 13. In fact, I was surprised that even five in that age group still relied on their natural eyesight ... though contact lenses probably lowered the count.

And here we come to an additional reason for seniors to wear glasses. Years ago I began to observe a phenomenon that for others may have gone unnoticed. As people age, their eyes seem to recede, appearing smaller and less obvious as a significant facial feature. Our eyeballs aren't actually getting any smaller, but they do drop back somewhat in the socket. Plus the skin around our eyes loses some of its plumpness and sags—just like other body parts.

During the years when I was still wearing contact lenses, I observed my own eyes becoming less distinctive. But wearing glasses brought them back to prominence again. So for both convenience and vanity I gave up the contacts in favor of an attractive frame around my eyes.

For us, the cosmetic importance of eyewear is demonstrated daily in the personage of Alex Trebek on *Jeopardy*. On his own program, with glasses, he is quite handsome. But nearly daily I've also seen him on CNN doing an insurance ad. There, with no glasses, he appears decidedly less handsome, certainly older.

CATARACTS ARE ANOTHER EYE DISORDER WHICH afflicts many seniors, but is easily remedied. Studies by the National Eye Institute show that, by age 80, more than half of all Americans either have a cataract or have had cataract surgery.

A cataract is a clouding of the lens in the eye. The lens is made of mostly water and protein. As we age, the protein may clump together, forming a "cloud" within the lens.

There are several factors, along with the wear and tear of age, that can contribute to the formation of cataracts, including health and environmental issues. Some of the early signs might be blurry vision, faded colors, poor night vision, and the appearance of a "halo" around lights.

Like most people our ages, Rob and I have undergone cataract surgery, first in one eye, then the other. Neither of us experienced any complications, which is the norm for this common procedure. We both enjoyed improved vision, though it's important to decide in advance among two possibilities—an improvement in distance vision versus close-up. Like many others, I opted for a different improvement in each eye. Rob chose dual visual acuity for close-up work ... meaning he wears glasses for distance vision, like driving.

According to the American Society of Cataract and Refractive Surgery, roughly three million Americans undergo cataract surgery each year, with an overall success rate of 98 percent.

Yet occasionally this surgery leaves the patient worse off, as happened with both my brother, Allan, and a good friend, Helen. Afterwards, both suffered double vision. But since Allan is an engineer, he was able to mathematically calculate how much his vision was "off," to report back to the surgeon, and have the problem corrected. He says he now sees perfectly.

Not so with Helen. Her double-vision has incapacitated her to such a degree that she had to give up driving, and she can no longer read comfortably, which would be devastating for bibliophiles like me. For her, audiobooks would be one answer.

Based on my brother's experience, I have urged her to have the lenses re-done, knowing from Allan that such correction is possible. But so far she agrees in principle, while not taking the steps to make it happen. Sadly, her quiet resistance is keeping her needlessly impaired.

AMONG THE SERIOUS THREATS TO VISION IS Macular Degeneration, which has no cure, but whose progress can be slowed by the lowering of eye pressures. Because one of my eyes shows some deterioration, my ophthalmologist is quite stern about keeping me on twice daily eye drops which lower internal pressure and slow the degenerative process. Though it's obvious to me that one eye sees less clearly than the other, I'm faithful about my drops and don't find the bad eye getting worse.

INEVITABLY, WE THINK BACK TO AN ERA WHEN ONLY inferior corrections were available to older folks whose vision deteriorated. It's comforting to know that, absent macular degeneration, our eyesight can be maintained throughout our lives—even very long lives.

And how about that other important window to the world—hearing. While the restorative news is not as promising as for vision, help is certainly available … as Rob and I both know.

CHAPTER EIGHT

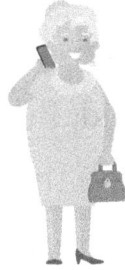

Tuning In, Or Tuning Out

ONE OF THE ADVANTAGES OF GETTING OLDER IS THE ability to blame hearing loss whenever you've deliberately tuned someone out. After nine decades of listening to people opine, my husband Rob has developed a knack for ignoring what other people are saying–especially the talking heads on television. He either pays scant attention to their words, or he puts the TV on mute and reads the captions at will. (For me, the text flows so fast across our screen, it's a challenge to read it all and grasp the meaning before it disappears.)

However, with Rob it's not just television. Even with hearing aids he has a difficult time with social conversation, missing large chunks of what is being said. But this may not be entirely due to hearing loss. Rob thinks most people talk too much, anyway, so his inability to discern every word of their dialogue hardly bothers him. He smiles and nods, but is blissfully willing to let large portions go unheard. I sense an attitude there. I guess you could say he's hard of hearing and he's heard enough.

NOT SO WITH ME. AS A WRITER AND ENTHUSIAST about social interactions, I'm disturbed that I miss so much of what people say. "What?" has become my habitual four-letter word. Yet constantly asking friends to repeat their comments can get annoying for all concerned, so I wear my hearing aids and listen intently—while I grudgingly accept that I may be missing out on conversational tidbits I really care about.

Rob's hearing is worse than mine. One of his ears

works so poorly that even his hearing aids do not bring it up to snuff. At home, we live with a largely unsolved problem: when I speak—almost incessantly, according to him—he tunes in mostly when he wants to.

The problem arises when he fails to answer—about half the time—so I'm left wondering which of my *very important words* he simply never heard. Of course the repercussions come later. "You never told me this," he says, which leaves an open issue … did I tell him about that dinner date, which he didn't hear, or have I forgotten whether I even said it?

It's comforting to know I'm not alone. A couple of years ago, on a book tour in a neighborhood far from mine, I was visiting with a dear friend whose name would be familiar to all of you. She introduced me to her very likable husband, but once we were in a different room where we couldn't be overheard, she said with a smile, "Milton is deaf in one ear. And he doesn't listen out of the other."

We both laughed. Later I found myself thinking,

Millions of people have listened to you avidly on radio and television, and laughed at your quips. Milton doesn't know what he's missing.

As with most couples, some issues hang like a winter coat in a California closet, neglected and its fate unresolved, for years. Both of us try for patience in such situations, but not always. One of us is patient, but feels she's often unfairly criticized, while the other is mostly impatient, never feels "hurt," but has an excellent memory. In a fair number of our back-and-forths, he maintains an air of superiority, meaning he knows he's right about the issue, so stop with the arguing already. Not being able to fully communicate because of hearing loss doesn't help matters. Perhaps as age lessens our ability to hear, we should focus on improving our ability to listen.

At least half the people in my age group have experienced significant hearing loss. It can lead to withdrawal from social activities which, in turn, may result in loneliness, depression, frustration and anger. All are negative emotions that can cause cognitive decline and poor health in other facets of life. If you are sitting at home in your recliner because you can't hear what people say, then you are not active and involved. I think it was Helen Keller who said, "Blindness cuts us off from things, but deafness cuts us off from people."

ON A LIGHTER NOTE, WE'VE HAD SOME FUNNY CONversations. I'm sure most readers have heard stories about the comical sequences that can arise from hearing problems. A typical one might go as follows:

Wife: "I hear that the Kennedys got a boat."

Husband: "Why would they do that, they don't even have a yard."

Wife: "They wouldn't put it in the yard, Honey, they'd keep it at the club."

Husband: "What do you mean? I don't know any clubs that would keep a goat."

Wife, suspiciously: "Did you put in your hearing aids?"

Husband: "No. I'm not wearing them. I didn't think there'd be anything important to hear today."

BY COINCIDENCE, JUST TODAY ROB AND I HAD OUR own peculiar conversation. We were sitting together on the edge of the bed when I looked behind us and said, "I'm trying to decide whose pillow is whose." At which he echoed me, or so he thought, "Which pair of shoes."

AND THUS WE GET TO HEARING AIDS.

Once again, Rob and I got ours at Costco, where the customer's hearing is thoroughly tested and the hearing aids tailored to his specific areas of loss. The appliances fall in a middle range of price, but the store offers free checkups and free replacement parts when something stops working. *If only Costco did hips and knees!*

My experience is that most hearing aids work better than no aids at all, but the end result is far from perfect. In a noisy room where lots of people are speaking, it's difficult to focus on one particular set of words. I can't count how many times I've laughed heartily at "something" a friend said while desperately hoping they weren't asking me a serious question.

Although all hearing aid companies swear they've solved the problem of background noise, the truth is, they haven't. And why would it seem reasonable to expect that one voice could ever be made to stand out from the jumble of others? It's like listening to a gaggle of geese. How does your personal hearing aid know exactly which goose you want to listen to?

What most of us rely on in a two-person exchange within a cocktail party atmosphere, are intense lip-reading and interpretation of facial expressions. You'll be out of luck if the other person has the pro-verbial poker face or a mouthful of hors d'oeuvres. Often enough we can hear the person's voice but are unable to distinguish their words. Thinking back, how often have I mouthed to someone, "I can't hear you!" Then with a directional nod, "Let's go over there, where it's quiet."

In fact, I wonder how much conversation is grasped even by the 20-somethings when they're in a noisy, crowded room. Many of our millennials

who've been present at a few thunderous concerts
soon begin to notice that their hearing has been
compromised ... inviting lectures from concerned,
older relatives—which they probably choose not to
hear.

I suspect that lots of wise seniors besides us are
alert to damage from loud noise and keen about
avoiding further loss. I, for one, am unwilling to
add preventable destruction to normal, age-related
deprivations. Whenever I'm caught in an overloud
situation from which I can't escape, I plug my ears.
And I don't care who notices.

Among science's many contributions to the
well-being of seniors, perhaps the biggest lag has
been in the area of age-related hearing loss. So far,
we all know the problem, but haven't yet found any
fool-proof solutions.

We can only hope that a few scientists, somewhere,
are out there, devoted to find hearing's equivalent to
vision's cataract surgery.

MEANWHILE, WE NEED TO LINGER, BRIEFLY, ON A subject vital to all of us in our 80s: how best to avoid falling down.

CHAPTER NINE

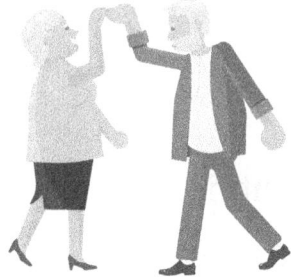

Staying Upright: Steady As She Goes

WHILE IT'S UNLIKELY THAT ANY OF US, LIKE HUMPTY Dumpty, will fall off a wall, it's possible that, as an eighty-year-old, you will eventually be the victim of a mild or serious spill. If so, we can only hope that the pieces, unlike those of an egg, can easily be put back together again.

If you think it can't happen to you, here's a few statistics from the CDC that might make you think again. One in four Americans aged 65 and above falls each year. Every 11 seconds, an older adult is treated in an emergency room for a fall. Every 19 minutes an older adult dies from a fall.

For any of us, a fall is pretty traumatic—even if it's within our own home and we happen to land on a padded rug.

The few falls I've taken really shook me up; each time, the whole episode felt scary, dangerous, and entirely out of control. Luckily I didn't hit any furniture on the way down. It's also fortunate that I inherited a large and extra strong skeleton. Since childhood my feet and hands have been huge, greatly beyond the norm ... which goes also for the accompanying, underlying structure. It took years before I fully appreciated how lucky I was that my heritage included a father who was a solid German with his own extra-strong skeleton.

Women with average, light frames are more prone than I am to breakage ... especially those suffering from the bone-thinning ailment called Osteoporosis. With a skeleton already somewhat compromised, a broken hip is too often the result of an accidental topple.

Unfortunately, long hospital confinements can be more dangerous than the original accident. We older humans don't fare well when we're bed-ridden for weeks on end. Not only do we lose physical conditioning, but we run the risk of thrombotic episodes, such as DVT (Deep Vein Thrombosis), PE (Pulmonary Emboli), or stroke.

Physicians try to prevent these events with medication and/or pressure equipment like elastic stockings.

But all good orthopedic surgeons recognize it's important for their patients to become ambulatory as soon as possible after any surgery, no matter what the age group.

THE GOOD NEWS IS THAT AWARENESS—FOLLOWED by prevention—is key to preventing accidents. Our family nurse, Lauren, a frequent witness to such problems, offers impromptu lectures on preventing falls. First, she says, get rid of all throw rugs, including those which sit atop a carpet, causing a height differential that can lead to stumbling. Even worse is the small rug that sits on a smooth surface and skids away under your feet. Either can eventually make a victim out of its owner. When she visits a patient's home, she isn't shy about ordering them to dispose of their throw rugs.

Second, she talks about junk that accumulates in a home's normal pathways.

Having both stumbled a few times over unexpected obstacles, Rob and I are acutely aware of leaving anything, anywhere, that invites a fall, especially in areas with limited lighting.

I once left a heavy box just inside our back door. It was then daylight, so I didn't think twice. But when I returned home after dark, I didn't see the impediment and flew over it and straight into our back porch freezer.

What a horrible surprise! But what an important—and luckily, damage-free lesson—that became. Ever since, I've been careful never to leave objects of any kind in or near our normal pathways. Both Rob and I are on constant patrol for heedlessly abandoned items. Our vigilance also helps to keep our home free of the clutter that so easily piles up over time.

Not all threats involve inanimate objects like boxes and throw rugs. You also need to be aware of an additional, self-induced hazard: the *risk of rushing*. Too often, being in a hurry is a prelude to disaster. We spin around too fast and lose our footing, we hurry past an obstacle but instead bump into it, we move so quickly up or down a few steps we don't sufficiently lift one foot or the other, and instead take a spill. When Rob sees me hurrying to accomplish something, he says, "Don't rush, Babe. Never rush. It's dangerous." And indeed, I am reminded of a friend who gathered her mail, changed direction suddenly, and fell into the street, suffering nasty injuries.

UNFORTUNATELY, WE HAVE MINIMAL, OR NO CONtrol over the environment outside our homes, which may help explain why so many of us walk with a slight stoop, always looking down to assess what obstacle might lie in our paths.

As we progress through parking lots we need to be aware of those four-inch barriers that define parking spaces ... and it's important to know when you might be close to stepping off a curb. Sadly, a longtime acquaintance recently died from the concussion he suffered after he fell off a curb and into the street.

In my daughter's home I'm constantly aware that various rooms are on different levels, and it's important to know when you're about to reach one of her many steps. The other day I said to Rob, "Tracy's home would never be purchased by anyone of an advanced age. He'd be in constant danger of forgetting about all those up and down steps."

Young people must have enhanced peripheral vision, because they so seldom fall over obstacles. I see kids skipping up sports bleachers without handholds, never looking down, but never stumbling, either.

In fact, not so many years ago I routinely ran up the stairs to my office, literally skipping steps as I went.

In what seemed like the blink of an eye, I realized my youthful nimbleness had abandoned me, and I suddenly needed a banister. Now I grip the railing, AND in the other hand, I maintain balance with a cane. It's obvious that carrying my teacup up those stairs is a challenge, now that both hands are occupied. If I need to transport something large, like a ream of paper, I place it down several steps ahead of me, and then, with repeated bend-overs, manage to move it, a few steps at a time, until it's carried to the top. It's slow going, but I'm pretty sure it counts as extra exercise—sort of like toe-touching, weight-lifting and a stair master all rolled into one.

THE STRANGEST FALL I EVER HAD DIDN'T INVOLVE any hazardous items to trip over or treacherous stairs to tumble down, but it easily could have resulted in serious, even permanent, damage. It happened about six years ago and began with a simple attempt to pick up a pair of theater tickets from our front porch. I was wearing new tennis shoes, never imagining they might pose a problem.

To this day it still mystifies me that such an innocent act could have escalated toward such a potential disaster. Somehow, as I straightened, I found I couldn't get my feet under me. The result was, I kept pedaling, trying to attain an upright position, but never quite succeeding.

Instead, all that leg work propelled me off the front porch, flying over two steps, and splatting onto our stone walkway. I landed hard on the rocks, scraping my wrist and leg and damaging a number of ribs. It was pure luck that my head never got involved.

Still, I knew I couldn't get to my feet. So I lay there screaming for Rob, who was sitting beyond the still-open front door, but now in his chair in the family room watching television.

For a long while he didn't hear my cries—and all because he happened to be watching the horrifying destruction of the space capsule *Challenger*. He thought those agonized cries were all coming from the TV.

Eventually, as I continued shouting (amazed that I had enough energy to yell), he realized some of the shouts were mine, and he hurried out to discover me lying helpless on the walkway.

"What happened, Babe?" he asked with plenty of concern. "How bad are you hurt? Can you get up?"

"I can't tell yet. But no, I can't get up. I can barely move."

He stood there, pondering. "Don't think I'm strong enough to pull you to your feet. I'll go call Chris."

Luckily for all of us, Chris, who lives nearby, was just arriving home from work, and he and Betty-Jo arrived within minutes.

"Do you still have your walker with a seat?" he asked, and it turned out we did—from one of our prior knee surgeries. I guess it's a good idea to hang onto your old medical equipment in case you need it again!

It took two of them to lift me onto the walker, and all three to carry the load up the two steps and into the house.

Once I was on the couch, Chris cleaned up various leg and wrist wounds, then examined my ribs. "They may be broken, Mom," he said, "but we don't do anything these days with cracked ribs. We just let them heal."

THE AMAZING AFTERMATH WAS THREE-FOLD: 1) X-rays showed my ribs were intact. 2) Two days later I gave a speech to a large senior audience, albeit sitting down. 3) I eventually figured out the reason I'd been unable to regain my balance while still on the porch: the new tennis shoes had extra-thick soles, which threw me off, so I never lifted my feet high enough to get them securely placed under me.

Needless to say, I sent them back for a full refund.

ONE REASON THAT FALLS REPRESENT SUCH A RISK for the aging is that they can be caused by a number of factors besides hazards in the environment. Among them are visual problems, physical frailty, a too-abrupt change of directions, and dizziness—the latter being an issue for Rob.

"Why are you having that problem?" I asked him one day.

"I'm really not sure about the cause, Babe. But several of my medications warn of dizziness as a side effect."

"Maybe you need anti-dizziness pills," I replied, wishing I had a better answer. For every pill, it seems, you need another pill to counteract the side-effects of the first pill.

FALLING IS NOT AN INEVITABLE CONSEQUENCE OF aging. There are practical lifestyle adjustments that can prevent you from ever taking a tumble. It is comforting to know that a variety of physical therapy facilities, private gyms and senior centers all offer exercises that can help prevent falls. The key is bolstering a senior's innate internal balance … part of which stems from small hairs in the inner ear, and part from strong leg muscles. After my front-porch fall, I spent hours in the gym. Among their routines were jaunts around the room tossing and catching a ball, walking across uneven surfaces, balancing on one leg, pedaling a stationary bike.

For years now—ever since that fall—I've spent a few minutes at bedtime (positioning myself between the bed and a bureau), balancing on one leg, then the other, each for a count of 80. I credit this routine with enabling me, on a few occasions, to recover from a stumble which might otherwise have sent me to the floor.

Sometimes I catch myself mentally complaining: *What a drag that I'm now stuck with all these bothersome tricks, just trying to stay even. All routines that no kid ever has to do. Oh, to be forty again.*

But hey, I decide later, *I'm still here, and except for tennis, skiing, and bike riding, still living the life I once led.*

So Bravo for Tricks!

EVEN AT EIGHTY AND ABOVE, THERE'S PLENTY OF good news in our lives. One of them is all about FOOD.

CHAPTER TEN

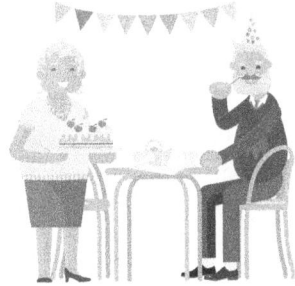

Let Them Eat Cake—But Not Quite So Much

I'VE LONG CONSIDERED MYSELF A HEALTH FOOD NUT. A health food nut who loves sweets.

Like other seniors our age, Rob and I are hell bent on keeping off the extra pounds, which is possible only by making adjustments in our everyday routines … and by this I don't mean "dieting."

Yet a study done several years ago by the Journal of American Medicine estimated that 70 percent of adults over the age of 60 are overweight or obese. Our metabolism changes as we age; we tend to exercise less and the muscle mass of our youth gets replaced by fat. But many seniors continue to eat the way they did when they were younger.

In recent years, Rob and I have made some significant changes that are helping us avoid the weight-gain pitfall.

And this, in spite of the fact I don't cook much anymore, falling back on an old excuse: *I've been there, done that.*

Way back when, I was cooking for six children (five boys and a girl), kids who were alike in many ways, but all with distinctive appetites. "Mom, you know I don't like my hamburger overdone," one would say, as opposed to the kid who complained, "Ugh, I can't eat this, Mom, it's practically raw." There was seldom any consensus on what constituted a great dinner.

Later I cooked for just Rob and me and sometimes I heard the same refrain: "You know I don't like zucchini," he noted, though I happened to love it. Whatever my accomplishments, praise seldom

followed me to the kitchen. So dinner-wise, I'm basically retired. But hey, in your 80s, you love it when
you're treated like a queen.

RETIRING FROM KITCHEN DUTY DOESN'T MEAN WE
eat out three times a day. I still make breakfasts, and
each day Rob squeezes fresh orange juice. Following
a routine partly created by him, he acts as if we're
governed by some mysterious, Otherworldly tradi-
tion. "It's Monday," he says, "we're due for Egg and
Toast." I'm fairly happy about Mondays and the easy-
to-make Egg and Toast.

But I'm also a fan of Creamed-Corn Omelets
and he isn't … which I push regularly, upping their
attractiveness by offering him an add-on, meaning
three slices of bacon.

Rob can count on a laugh when he refers to *"the
dreaded corn omelet."*

Unrelenting force or not, we've set up a loose
schedule for our day's first meal (i.e. egg sandwich on
Tuesday, whole-wheat pancakes on Friday), that Rob

seems determined to follow, lest there be a penalty for going off course. If that isn't *rigid*, it comes close.

Yet here's where we vary from younger members of the Wills clan; we eat only two meals a day ... which are all we want. The first comes in late morning, between ten and twelve, the last around five or six.

We allow ourselves a midday snack of nuts or a cup of yogurt, (in my case, sometimes a stealthy trip to the freezer for one See's candy. *Out of sight, out of mind* ensures you don't eat five in one day. Besides, it takes time to eat a frozen chocolate.)

The good news is, Rob weighs about 20 pounds fewer than he did some dozen years ago, and I've dropped to my college weight, though with a different distribution. (The original was better).

The truth must be that we're simply not eating as much as we once did; it seems that both of us tend to fill up quicker. In addition, I, for one, am drawn each day to exercise ... namely, I read student manuscripts or the newspaper as I pedal my stationary bike.

Over the years we've found that tricks-for-the-

Eighties are everywhere, and meals are just another example. While the two of us pretty much eat what we want and never feel deprived, we've also learned ways to make it all work.

FOR DINNER, ROB AND I ARE OFTEN INVITED TO EAT with one or the other of our kids, two of whom live nearby. We get regular invitations from our daughter and her Paul, or we're asked to sup with son Chris and wife Betty-Jo. Both families tend to serve meals that would suit most experts on nutrition. Always low-fat meats or fish, always a vegetable or salad, few desserts. But for us, small portions. They've caught on, as we have, that we now have smaller appetites.

Though Rob and I have reduced our overall calorie intake, we are always on the lookout for a dessert, so both households tend to ply us with ice cream. But these days it's only one scoop.

WITHIN THESE GENERALITIES, WE ARE STRICT ABOUT some foods: We always buy whole grain breads, we stick to organic eggs from free-range chickens, plus organic milk (from cows not fed hormones). And we avoid anything sweetened with high fructose corn syrup. Our primary supplier tends to be Costco ... which also offers great pre-cooked choices for those rare occasions when we have our second meal at home.

During our frequent dinners in fast-food or modest restaurants, we each have our favorite items. Yet we often agree to go for fish at H Salt ... or a hamburger at In 'n Out. I'm aware that their buns are made with white flour and probably not worth much as a nutrient. I can only hope that the abundant lettuce and tomatoes add value that the bread lacks.

In addition, the Boston Market chain offers a complete, nutritious, and inexpensive meal. We've noticed it's a favorite among all age groups.

Our weekly routine includes Soup Plantation, where both of us load up on veggies. For that one day, at least, we're dining at the top of the nutrition scale.

Only about once or twice a month—always with

friends or family—do Rob and I treat ourselves to dinner at high-end restaurants. What's not to like about a selection of great entrees and enough leftover food for dinner the next day?

Yet we never seem drawn to fancy eateries when it's just *us*. For Rob and me, cost is one factor, but even more is the time consumed by "fine dining."

Rob is apt to say, "I've got to get home, Babe. I have a lot of TV to watch." As with breakfasts, in our house there's something almost sacred about *established routine*, about making sure we see two news programs, plus each night's *Jeopardy* plus BBC dramas, plus Sunday's *Sixty Minutes*.

God forbid that we should ever be out of touch with world events.

I REALIZE THAT MANY SENIORS IN OUR AGE GROUP reside in assisted-living facilities with full room and board. Since I've enjoyed lunches or dinners at numerous high-end group homes in the course of giving speeches about writing, it's been obvious that their meals had the benefit of dietary and nutritionist input. In every case the food was delicious; clearly there was no need for grocery shopping.

THESE DAYS I MAY BE SPENDING LESS TIME IN THE kitchen but, like Rob, am governed by habits—which apply equally to food.

Aware that for some reason I'm almost never thirsty (and hearing zealots preach about the need for hydration), my morning begins with a full—and forced—glass of water, accompanied by the attitude, *There, I got that over with.*

Also, there's a mantra that sometimes runs through my head—*don't forget the nuts!* Ever since I was the "with" author on a book by Dr. John West, a breast-care surgeon, his section on nutrition has helped govern our eating habits. The doctor reports that he often asks his patients, "Which food do you think is most associated with longevity?"

Invariably the patient replies, "broccoli."

"Not broccoli," says my doctor. "It's nuts."

"Really? Nuts? Aren't they fattening?"

"That doesn't seem to matter," says my doctor. "And any nuts will do—even peanuts." Next he says, "I eat a small handful every day. They make a filling snack between meals."

Thus, Rob and I keep handy a jar of mixed, unsalted nuts. But to make up for no salt, we add raisins. We can only hope the longevity Dr. West mentions means years and not months.

AND SPEAKING OF LONGEVITY ... ROB AND I ARE fortunate that we never smoked. As teenagers, we each had a parent who discouraged us from even trying—especially Rob's father, who made his son sign a no-smoking pledge etched on wood.

Also, unlike others in our age group for whom an evening cocktail hour is a must, Rob and I never drink at home; we simply never get around to it.

I once bought a six-pack of beer as a sleep aid, and six months later realized I'd forgotten to drink even one.

Health experts offer conflicting advice on whether a daily drink is good or bad.

While Rob and I often have one cocktail apiece when we're out with friends or family, a second drink never seems appealing. In this, we're probably just lucky, or maybe intuitively cautious. Both of us had close relatives who were alcoholics.

THOUGH MANY A NUTRITIONIST CLAIMS A WELL-rounded diet requires no supplemental vitamins, they're advocating so many fruits and vegetables that to get enough you'd have to be gulping them down all day long. So Rob and I both take a daily multivitamin recommended for our ages, plus additional Lutein (for eyes), and extra "C" and "D".

A last comment about food: the experts can't seem to agree on the value of coffee. One moment it's touted as great for your health, especially if you manage to gulp down three or four cups a day. The next it comes with caveats. For Rob, coffee is a necessary adjunct to breakfast, giving him the energy to start his day. ("My drug of choice," he says.)

Not so for me. More than a few swallows gives me a stomach ache. Instead, I drink green tea sweetened with Stevia. And most days that's it.

But not always. Sometimes when I plan to spend the day writing, I add an additional tea bag to my cup—meaning English Breakfast tea with its extra punch. It turns out I'm a lot smarter on black tea than green.

Yet the caveats continue: *smarter* only happens when it's occasional. As with all stimulants, the beneficial effect lessens when they're used on a regular basis.

LIKE MANY A CAFFEINE—SENSITIVE PERSON, I MAKE it a point never to drink tea past four in the afternoon. Any later and falling asleep would be impossible. Frankly, it's a wonder to me that older Brits manage to sleep at all … so many of them enjoy that late-afternoon, heavily caffeinated tea ritual.

During our many trips to the British Isles, Rob and

I became enamored of their engaging tea-times and all their little biscuits. But we were mostly young then, and sleep came easily.

WHICH REMINDS ME—THE IMPORTANCE OF SLEEP IS just now blooming in American magazines and on the news. Thus the next chapter is all about certain tricks ... about why, when, and how to sleep.

CHAPTER ELEVEN

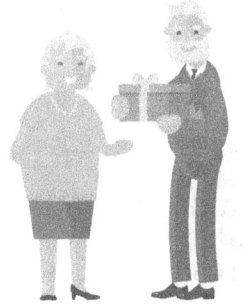

Sleep: The Important Third of Your Life

SLEEP DENIERS HAVE A PAT PHRASE: "I'LL CATCH UP on my rest when I die."

What they don't know is, by denying their bodies essential sleep, they're hastening the day when their Eternal Rest will begin.

Perhaps this attitude began with rock musician Warren Zevon who, in a 1976 song title, coined the well-known idiom, "I'll sleep when I'm dead."

Zevon, by the way, died at the rather young (from

my perspective), age of 56.

The following excerpt comes from a book titled, *WHY WE SLEEP, Unlocking the Power of Sleep and Dreams*, by Matthew Walker, PhD. This paragraph, a direct quote from the book, imagines the public's response if these were the lead sentences in a news story:

AMAZING BREAKTHROUGH!

Scientists have discovered a revolutionary new treatment that makes you live longer. It enhances your memory and makes you more creative. It makes you look more attractive. It keeps you slim and lowers food cravings. It protects you from cancer and dementia. It wards off colds and the flu. It lowers your risk of heart attacks and stroke, not to mention diabetes. You'll even feel happier, less depressed, and less anxious. Are you interested?

The magic is that all these marvelous results can

be achieved without drugs, therapies, or medical miracles. All you have to do is get enough sleep. Throughout the book the author cites numerous studies to back up this one paragraph.

I have now read the entire volume, but already knew from my own experience that the tenets of this paragraph are true.

From a thorough examination of this long essay, plus articles consumed and speeches heard over the years, I recognized that the hours spent sleeping are analogous to putting your car in the shop for a thorough examination and replacement of worn parts. During those hours, and through several stages of sleep, rejuvenation of the brain and repairs to multiple bodily systems (for example, the immune system), take place in ways that aren't possible when you're awake.

Most of us wouldn't be pleased by a mechanic who said, "If you give me a few hours today, I can fix parts of your car. But frankly, I don't have time to do a thorough job. You'll just have to take your chances that it won't stall on the freeway. Or you can come back some other time. Whenever."

That would be enough to send you scrambling to find a different mechanic. But with your own body you have choices. You can do whatever it takes to attain a good night's sleep, or you can postpone the repair job and just "take your chances."

YEARS AGO, WHEN I WAS AT STANFORD TAKING exams, I deduced from past experience that I'd do better with fewer hours of late-night studying and more such hours tucked in bed.

Next day, with my mind alert, I could often conjure up a mental picture of where on the textbook page the needed words appeared. From there, with some "boring in," the answer had a way of popping onto my mental screen, almost magically.

This isn't to say I got straight "A's." I didn't. But my years at Stanford, and later UCLA, proved to my own satisfaction the huge benefits derived from hours spent snoozing. Also, in my experience through living many years, no other single route to happiness and a modicum of success, can equal being alert and "feeling good."

Aware of its importance in my life, I've striven to make getting enough rest a priority. But marriage, and then raising six kids, were significant impediments to attaining that "nicely energized" state. I was often so tired I didn't feel like doing anything. Always wary about artificial boosts to energy, for me taking "uppers" never seemed an answer. Instead it seemed wiser to take a nap … or head for bed a little earlier.

Back in our child-rearing days, I annoyed my rarin'-to-go husband so much that he complained, "All you care about is sleep."

Now that Rob, at age 92, regularly drops off while watching television, he's stopped repeating that refrain.

FOR YEARS I TOOK THE OCCASIONAL SLEEPING PILL, often furnished by my doctor-father, who was then president of Winthrop Laboratories. When Rob and I visited him in Port Washington, he was apt to take me aside and ask, "Maralys, do you need a sleeping pill?"

Usually I didn't, but he gave them to me anyway. And what a night's sleep the occasional Lotusate provided! It was probably best that this didn't happen often.

Mostly, with enough exercise and other sleep-conducing factors, for years pills weren't part of our routine—either Rob's or mine.

But then, abruptly, things changed. Like so many other seniors, we both began experiencing insomnia, with frequent wake-ups throughout the night. For this, my doctor was willing to prescribe low-dosage sleeping pills.

Then, during this 80s decade, things changed again. It seems the problem no longer resides with *falling asleep*. For me, with a modicum of daily exercise, that part has become easy. The tricky thing is *getting back to sleep* once you've been awake enough to make the inexorable trip to the bathroom.

So I've adjusted. I now take my sleeping pill after a

few hours, mainly when I'm on the way back to bed.

Also, I alternate pills, on an every-other-night basis. Both my internist and rheumatologist are okay with this. I suppose they've decided that a patient in her eighties may be a tad dependent … but who cares?

PEOPLE IN OUR AGE GROUP NEED EVERY ADVANTAGE for getting a good night's sleep, starting with establishing a set time when possible and customizing the sleep environment.

Most physicians suggest setting up a bedtime routine, such as phasing out strenuous activity and high-intensity television entertainment. They also recommend avoiding cell phones, computers, and late evening meals, not to mention forgoing stimulants like caffeine and chocolate.

The bedroom environment should include a bed with desired softness, a pillow geared to individual preferences, plus elimination of almost all sources of light.

Studies have shown that sleep is deeper when light

is eliminated.

There seems to be a difference of opinion regarding dead silence versus "white noise." We have long used a background fan, usually an air filter, as a gentle hum in the bedroom. Actually, an air filter may have benefits besides supplying "white noise."

Temperature in the bedroom is also a factor to consider. Most experts recommend the lower range of room temperatures, which would mean the high 60s. There is probably a tendency for most bedrooms to be kept too warm.

Finally, the matter of sleep is so important at any age, but particularly in our advanced years, that problems of sleep should be discussed with a personal physician or, in more serious cases, with a geriatric specialist.

IN SPITE OF ALL WE KNOW ABOUT THE FACTORS THAT lead to restful sleep, there are times when we oldsters wake up prematurely, often near dawn, aware that we're still tired, but unable to resume slumbering …

when even the nightly sleeping pill has worn off, yet we can't come up with a decent alternative.

Instead we're apt to defeat additional rest by trying to solve problems, or pondering a conflict, or reviewing the next day's to-do list. Pretty soon our thoughts are spinning like a hamster on his wheel. Misguided musing, at best.

For that, Rob and I have different remedies: he simply lies very still, tries not to arouse his mental state, and more often than not manages after awhile to drift off once more.

None of that works for me, the list-prone German. Instead, I push my chore-list aside and deliberately focus on a fruits-and-vegetable list, starting with "A" for asparagus and artichokes, and ending with "Z" for zucchini. If I'm lucky, I don't get past "M" for Mango. Or sometimes I recite countries, starting with "A" for Australia, or boys' names, starting with Anthony.

None of these strategies works all the time, especially if I've been so careless as to consume some late-night stimulant, like that stealthily-consumed chocolate.

FOR MOST OF US, THEN, THE SLEEP DISRUPTIONS that ensue with intercontinental travel are sufficient evidence that sleep, or the lack of it, can negatively influence your productivity and especially your outlook on life. Upsetting your body's natural circadian rhythm—your internal clock—can cause fatigue, impaired concentration, gastrointestinal problems and mood swings. When somebody complains, "Forgive me, but I'm jet-lagged," we all understand what he means. With that he gets a pass on grouchy or perplexing behavior.

WITH THIS THOUGHT IN MIND, THE NEXT CHAPTER describes some necessary tricks for enduring and minimizing the hassles of long-distance travel.

CHAPTER TWELVE

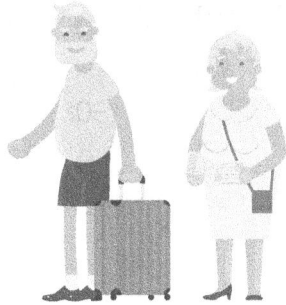

Getting There *Used To Be* Half the Fun

OH, FOR THAT LITTLE QUIVER OF EXCITEMENT WE all once knew! When, with bags packed, we barreled down a fast-moving road or freeway, paused briefly in an airport, and easily boarded a welcoming, seat-spacious plane.

In those days, front or back didn't much matter. With plenty of room for our legs, even in coach, with the certainty of a delicious en-route meal, with the help of young, cheerful, and rested flight attendants ready to bring us whatever extras we needed, even champagne, getting there really *was* half the fun.

Back then the plane's restrooms were decent size, roomy enough so you could actually turn around. If you needed to change clothes into something comfier, less formal, you could. Besides, people usually came on board dressed in their nicest, spiffiest best. After all, we were about to be *seen*. *Observed*. Who among us wanted to come off looking like a slob?

Nobody. Or at least that's what I remember.

TODAY, TRAVEL ISN'T HALF THE FUN. OR EVEN A quarter of the fun. In fact, it's mostly, but not always, hellish.

Start with the freeways—to wherever. Once a quick way to travel regionally, such trips have taken a depressing, downward turn. If we don't allow for traffic that often moves about thirty miles an hour and multiply that by the miles, we set ourselves up to miss the plane. No one, at any age, needs that kind of stress. Airport transport services insist that we allow an extra hour—or maybe two—now that flow of traffic matters more than distance.

Then there's the airport itself … and never mind fussing about the parking. It's considered crazy to take your own car, at least for a trip of a week or more.

Once inside most big-city airports, even if check-in moves quickly, we can count on a major, aerobic-exercise hike. Check-in is seldom anywhere close to TSA.

"But I didn't plan to walk for half an hour," I heard myself moaning as we traversed England's Heathrow. Still, for the young and exercise-prone, a long, pre-flight stroll may be an advantage. Once settled in his confined coach seat, the young traveler probably won't be able to move at all—or even, possibly, cross his legs.

But hey … with TSA now firmly in place between us and the plane, the nasty aspects are far from finished: next follows a long, no-chairs line. Then comes the undressing: jacket off, shoes off … and God forbid if your bra is suddenly showing, or you've got holes in your socks. (Way back when, I never took *anything* off. My dress-up clothes stayed right where they were.)

At best, the TSA line moves quickly and they didn't find anything suspicious in your carry-on ... meaning even your toothpaste or shampoo bottle needs to contain no more than three ounces.

There are exceptions for liquid medications over the three-ounce limit, but they vary by country, so you need to check with the airline regarding these. The Air Carrier Access Act requires airlines to allow various medical devices and aids, like collapsible wheelchairs and canes, to be carried on without counting them against your two-bag limit. Generally, that also includes CPAP machines and portable oxygen, but most airlines ask travelers to notify them ahead of time if they are bringing such items.

If you are new to traveling and seeing the world is on your "hoped-for" list, don't risk spoiling the trip by not knowing what you can't bring on board a plane— like anything flammable, explosive, or chemical, as well as knives, guns and those gel insoles that keep your tired feet from aching. Yes, those are banned and should be packed in your checked luggage.

And speaking of guns, with all this well-publicized scrutiny, it's hard to fathom why more and more Americans are currently stopped because their smallish suitcase, now traveling on the conveyer belt toward X-ray, inexplicably includes a gun. Which, TSA reports, is most often loaded!

We've all seen the photos on television: rows and rows of confiscated handguns, every make and size, taken from supposedly-innocent travelers. Most of them cry in dismay, "I forgot it was there!"

One can't help wondering—*when you packed your gun, back there in your bedroom, why didn't you pause as you added other items to your carry-on? Did you think, perhaps, that buried under your hair dryer, the gun might go unnoticed?*

Unfortunately, as TSA is loath to admit, the odd weapon does get past the examiner and travels with its owner in the passenger cabin. The rest of us are lucky that since 9/11, none of those guns have been used.

FROM CARRY-ON INSPECTION LINES TO BOARDING gate, the distance is often agreeably short. Still, a quick glance at fellow passengers makes it plain that this is anything but a special occasion. Instead, it appears we're all headed for a backyard barbecue. Nobody seems excited or even anticipatory.

Almost everyone wears jeans, sweatpants and athletic shoes ... sometimes even flip-flops. Tee-shirts outnumber collared shirts. I once saw a young lady boarding a plane in what appeared to be her pajamas. Messy hair and an absence of makeup suggests even the women don't care much how they look; did they, perhaps, tumble out of bed and rush to the airport without a glance in the mirror?

With arms already full, almost everyone is also pushing a wheeled case, some so gigantic you wonder, *Will that thing fit in the overhead compartment?*

And soon begins what all those passengers hope

for, but few achieve—arrival at a seat where he or she can repose comfortably for the length of the flight … a perch free of overlappers. A site where it's possible to stretch or change positions.

Too bad, folks. Today, in the coach section of most planes (except for those few rows with roomier seats, for which the passenger pays extra—or the exit rows), such seats are no longer standard.

Unfortunately, most airlines have garnered extra profit by reconfiguring their cabin interiors, cramming the once-reasonable passenger space with extra rows of seats.

It's only fair to admit that one huge improvement makes travel markedly better: we're no longer breathing cigarette smoke.

Otherwise, it's too bad for anyone who still yearns for the Good Old Days, when *Getting There Was Half the Fun.*

WITH ALL THIS GRIM NEWS COMES A FEW BRIGHT spots for the seniors among us. With certain tricks, parts of this scenario can be upgraded.

To start, the remedy for Too Much Traffic is allowing yourself Too Much Time. When you know you'll make the plane for sure, sitting in slow-moving traffic isn't so nerve-wracking.

Once at the airport, or sometimes when you buy your ticket, you can ask for a wheelchair. While for Rob and me this once hurt our pride, in recent years the wheelchair request has been a godsend. Most airports are good about furnishing this kind of help, which goes beyond mere transportation.

Not only does some cheerful person push you for miles (or so it seems), but they're gracious about stopping, and helping, at kiosks that deal with TSA PreCheck or Global Entry.

If you travel often, paying an extra $85 for five years of TSA PreCheck, or $100 for five years of Global Entry, will help expedite your passage through security—and you won't have to remove your little bag of liquids or small electronics

Once at TSA, most of us get additional special

treatment. We are whisked past long lines, and in the U.S., at least, we don't have to remove our shoes, belts, or light jackets.

That helpful person also lifts our carry-ons onto the conveyor belt, and we are asked to stand only briefly, while going through the X-ray machine. Still, if it happens that we have artificial knees or hips, and we set off an alarm, we are soon examined in more detail, literally patted down.

And here we want to protest that TSA examiners, as a group, have gotten an undeserved bad rap. During our many trips, at least in the U.S., neither of us has ever had a bad experience. Almost all such people have been efficient, courteous, and pleasant to deal with. We tend to see so many smiles and so much good will, that we often end up thanking them.

We assume that it's usually that stereotypical "Ugly American" who ends up bleating about his bad TSA treatment—the kind of person who picks fights everywhere he goes.

IT'S IMPORTANT TO NOTE THAT THE SAME KIND OF helpfulness occurs when we request wheelchairs in Amsterdam, London, or Paris. In fact some of these airports are so huge we wonder how anyone of any age is fit enough to hike those vast distances ... which can add up to a couple of miles.

But then, most people in Europe—in fact in a lot of countries besides ours—tend to walk a great deal more than we do. In general, during our various out-of-country trips we've seen far less obesity than here in the United States. Too many of us are hell bent on getting around in ways that don't include our legs.

A LAST TRICK THAT HELPS PROVIDE A PLEASANT TRIP by air: If you can afford it, choose Business or First Class. As a retired senior, your schedule may be flexible enough for you to travel midweek days and avoid holiday weekends. Airline fares vary widely; knowing this, most of us aim for a Tuesday, Thursday, or Saturday, when fares are lowest.

In the past, Rob and I were able to buy a coach

ticket and ensure an upgrade with miles; it worked every time. Unfortunately, the miles upgrades on many airlines are rapidly disappearing.

American Airlines, for one, is so bent on saving their best seats for full-fare passengers, that it's only a stroke of luck if you manage to find a Business Class seat that's not already taken. Still, sometimes it happens.

The two of us are now so uncomfortable in coach that we refuse to travel more than a few hours in one of those ever-narrower seats. For us, it's no longer the lack of food that matters (with free meals for trips fewer than six hours no longer offered in back), it's the agonizing lack of seat, leg, and shoulder room. It's having a stranger's arm intruding into your personal space, or their head scant inches from yours. It's the requirement that you sit for hours drawn in upon yourself in a kind of pre-natal position.

For someone whose weight is under 140, coach might be an option. For us, neither markedly over-weight but taller than average, traveling like this means we'd rather not go.

And here's the irony: Even First Class, on some airlines, with some flights, has become ever closer to the space allotment, food-quality, and rest-room size that were once offered in coach.

On a recent First Class flight on Alaskan Airlines, the cabin was so cold I found myself shivering, regretting that I hadn't thought to bring a jacket. Although the flight attendant said the captain would warm up our area, nothing ever changed. Finally I asked, "Do you have a blanket, or pillow?"

"Not up here," she said. "I'll check in back." Moments later she returned. "Sorry. No blankets or pillows."

"On this whole plane?" I asked.

She shrugged apologetically. "Nothing."

The hours became an exercise in endurance, as I forced my mind away from the cold and onto other issues.

Later, when I related the experience to my daughter, she said, "Mom, I learned long ago that you have to bring a warm jacket onto a plane. Always. You never know what the cabin temperature will be. I've learned my lesson."

Well, so have I. Still, it's hard to believe that a reputable airline like Alaskan would not equip their first class section with a few blankets and pillows. Or for that matter, the same for the people in back.

All of us can only wish that there was more competition and more airlines to choose from.

AS YOU PREPARE FOR A TRIP BY PLANE, IT'S HELPFUL to remember that we are all inclined to over-pack; we bring clothes or other items that we never use. Aware of this, the most experienced travelers tend to carry the least.

As to suitcases, Rob and I now require luggage with four spinner wheels rather than two roller wheels. It's easier to push than pull—especially when we stack one bag on top of another.

OF COURSE FOR SENIORS, DRIVING OR GOING BY

train are additional options. We can't speak for long-distance train travel, but we suppose that if time is of no importance, that might be the best and easiest way to travel … though a friend reports that even the trains are now downgraded.

However, we've noticed that locally all our freeways are increasingly crowded, and for ever-longer periods of time. With some there's no longer a "rush-hour." It's all non-rush, from morning to late at night.

It goes without saying that a trip by road requires a comfortable car with good tires, brakes, and sound system.

Here we issue a caution about neighborhood travel: more and more we've observed that even after our light has turned green, one or two cars crossing in front of us have chosen to act on the yellow caution light by speeding up, thus sailing through on the red. If you've started immediately into the intersection, you're in trouble.

Before we enter on a new green, Rob and I look in both directions, just making sure that the intersection has cleared; God help you if you happen to jump in early, and someone else is crossing late.

Which brings us to a new trick for the older years. Quite a few of us senior couples find it's easiest to drive together, as pairs. On this topic, the next chapter will be short, but presumably helpful.

CHAPTER THIRTEEN

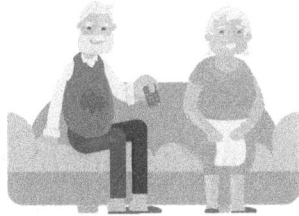

Team Driving

IT'S NOT BY ACCIDENT THAT ALL AIRLINES REQUIRE two pilots in the cockpit. With an airplane full of people, it's vital that the aircraft have supplementary and backup control.

In fact, in our country, pilots are given assertiveness training classes, just to make sure that the non-dominant pilot feels free to speak up when something goes wrong. A second brain can sometimes perceive what the first one missed.

As a vivid illustration, we know of one Korean

airline accident which occurred at SFO (San Francisco International Airport) because in the pilots' home country the primary pilot is held in such high esteem that the co-pilot feels he dares not question the other's judgment. As a result, the plane came in too low and hit a barrier before it reached the runway. A subsequent National Transportation Safety Board investigation revealed that the co-pilot knew their approach was wrong, but Korean protocol forbade his shouting an alarm. Fortunately, the death toll was lower than it might have been.

This very scenario was predicted by a member of the NTSB who helped me write a techno-thriller about a villain who decided to sabotage airplanes. In the years since *Scatterpath* was published, in 1993, every one of my expert's dire predictions about possible airline disasters has come true. Each involved preventable mistakes and produced significant fatalities. A history like that leaves an indelible impression about the steps needed in your own life to avoid accidents.

As older couples, we and some of our friends have agreed it is wise to drive as a team. Sometimes this is a spoken agreement, sometimes only a tacit understanding. But most of us recognize the importance of a second pair of eyes in the cockpits of our cars. One such couple calls itself, "Team Martin."

A host of factors make driving more difficult as we age: Vision and hearing problems, stiff joints and muscles that make it hard to turn your head, slower reaction time and reflexes, and even some medications. Any one of these can impair driving. In fact, the National Institute on Aging recommends that seniors avoid driving altogether when bad weather or traffic conditions make it more hazardous.

In some areas, organizations like AARP and AAA offer defensive driving classes for seniors, and likewise, some insurance companies offer discounts when the course is completed.

The need to double team became obvious to Rob and me one night on our way home from the music center. He was about to turn right onto a major highway, but his head was pointed left to make sure the way was clear. It was, and he began to pull out.

Before he'd gone far I shouted, "Stop! A bicycle!"

Reacting quickly, he braked. And there, crossing in front of us from the right was a man pedaling away, oblivious to our presence. Without my shout, he would have ended up on our hood.

Rob's assumption that it was safe to turn would normally have been okay. It was late in the evening, when no driver would expect anyone to be riding a two-wheeler in a nowhere part of town.

"Thanks, Babe!" Rob said. "You saved us!"

Since that day, the two of us have agreed that we're better off driving with each other. The fact is, Rob is usually at the wheel, but he curbs his normal impatience when I issue a warning that really wasn't needed.

And I, as a consequence, try to remain alert to possible hazards he might not see … without squealing every time another car gets too close.

It's a delicate balance, both for our safety and our

marriage. A little supportive teamwork on the road has kept us out of the ditch and out of divorce court.

ONCE YOU'VE REACHED AN AGE WHEN YOU'RE NO longer innovating new ways to conduct your life, your days can be smoother if you form good habits and let yourself off a few hooks.

CHAPTER FOURTEEN

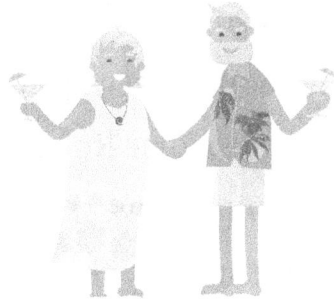

Making Habits Work For You

I NEVER WASTE TIME LOOKING FOR MY CAR KEYS.

Since, like other familiar objects, you have to put them *somewhere*, I routinely keep the keys in a special section of my purse. It's a habit that serves me well. Simply carrying my bag to the car will ensure I'll be able to start it.

Not everything in mine or my husband's life works this smoothly. The worst issue for me (and sometimes Rob), is the piece of paper that I set down someplace on my way to someplace else. I've squandered hours of time, cumulatively, searching for a document that I *know* must be in a limited space between say, the family room doorway and the kitchen. The problem here is that neither Rob nor I have developed a default spot for *temporary set downs.* Thus we've ensured we'll be victimized by these infuriating searches.

On the other hand, some behaviors are so habitual, so automatic, that they leave no trace in our brains and we can't decide later whether we actually did them. *Did I for instance, actually shake a little Stevia into my teacup?* All too often, I've done it but never noticed. Increasingly, as the years pass, these perfunctory tasks escape our memory. Friends have remarked, "I sometimes return home after a few miles to see if I remembered to close the garage door."

AS WE CONTINUE TO AGE, LIFE THROWS US MORE AND more small chores that we must do on a regular basis—or find ourselves forgetting them altogether. Some I've relegated to habit, others not.

Among the *habits that help* are the floor exercises

I call my "Huff and Puffs." They can be done any old time of day, but I've lately decided they're best performed as we watch our nightly *Jeopardy!* Since I'm unlikely to come up with more than three answers (which I can call out from the floor), it's become a habit to get out the exercise pad and stretch-away as the show progresses. Rob knows the personal interviews are my preferred moment, so he helps me time my viewing so I'm sitting up straight when Trebek interviews the players.

Similarly, I've long used the moments before bedtime to stand between bed and bureau for my one-legged balance exercises. These would surely be forgotten if I hadn't turned them into a nightly ritual. Likewise, those neck stretches (now consuming about one minute), have become part of each day's shower. Once in bed, I automatically put glaucoma drops in my eyes. And my first task each morning as I reach the kitchen is to drink a glass of water.

Yet my eyes' daytime drops have never become habitual—thus, too often, I forget them.

Other habits are doubtless common with everyone: you buckle your seat belt before the car leaves your street, you brush your teeth before bedtime and you stand on the scale (at your lightest), first thing in the morning. You probably take your pills—as we do—at a certain time of day, depending on whether they're designated for before or after meals.

Furthermore, we all tend to keep our pills in a pre-assigned spot … god help us if we had to waste time on periodic pill-searches.

Still, daily living affords endless ways to enlist rituals as automatic reminders. Back in my college days, I let my wardrobe pile up on the floor as I discarded each day's garments. Eventually this required a monumental day of reckoning. No longer. Once married, I hung up or put away each item as I took it off … which means for years there's been no trauma involved in choosing an outfit—or even dressing in a hurry.

Much as I've tried to persuade Rob to adopt a similar pattern, he remains a piler-upper … and a large part of what he takes off ends up on the floor. He insists he knows where everything is, though for me it would take some kind of topographical map.

Consequently, our dressing room has its neat and messy sides, as if a smart bomb targeted only half the room. But even here there's a habit involved: you can't maintain a long marriage with constant nagging. Some battles must be lost, graciously, in favor of marital harmony.

The losing issues you sometimes feel you can't endure ... well, you end up talking to yourself and deciding which does you the biggest favor—trying to get your own way, or opting to overlook and ignore the long-term, relatively unimportant matters.

Don't Sweat the Small Stuff ... and it's all small stuff, was a best-selling book two decades ago and the admonishment is never more relevant than after you've been married as long as we have—seventy years. When your relationship is new you argue about silly things like lights left on or off, what to watch on television, whether to run the air-conditioner, or when to go to bed. By the time you are in your 80s and have shared ups and downs, joys and sorrows, and seen your children become grandparents, life's mundane tribulations become much less important and your days are full of compromises.

THE LONGER YOU LIVE, THE MORE YOU NOTICE THAT the hours are flying by at an ever faster pace, and you'd better "double up" on unavoidable chores. Thus, because I have so many books and articles I want to read (plus my student manuscripts), it seems prudent to read as I pedal my stationary bike. This fulfills two priorities at once—exercise, plus reading-for-enjoyment, or editing those manuscripts. For the latter, I stop pedaling momentarily so I can write comments on my students' work.

Come to think of it, even today's shower includes a second long-standing habit—the cleansing of fingernails under the strongest portion of the hot water torrent.

Occasionally, I use the shower for a third

purpose—enhancing creativity. I'm not the only author who has noticed that a shower seems to open up your mind, bringing words and well-crafted sentences cascading into your thoughts, thus solving many a writing problem. Unable to jot anything down, I keep these valuable words from escaping by repeating them over and over until I'm out again and dry.

AS I MULLED OVER THIS TOPIC, IT BECAME CLEAR that habits seem to follow us wherever we go, and most are good; they lessen confusion and eliminate chaos, both hazardous to your sense of well-being.

For instance, when I check into a hotel, or settle into a suite on a ship, I decide, without much thought, where I'll store my suitcase or extra shoes, where I'll put my eye drops, which end of the closet will be Rob's and which mine. The alternative would be to dump everything into the middle of the room, where we'd both have to work around the mess.

Another predictable habit occurs regularly in my

classroom. It seems that wherever a student chooses, seemingly by accident, to sit on the first day of class, that seat becomes his for the rest of the semester. It's one of those mysterious, but oft-witnessed behaviors.

Rob says the same holds true for lawyers who choose their seats at the beginning of a deposition. When someone varies from this ritual, the original owner complains, "That's my seat," as though the spot was pre-assigned to him by some superior, unseen power.

Come to think of it, in my various groups where we regularly meet, each of us always sits in the same place. It would feel like stealing to take over someone else's spot.

Some of my students have been taking my class for years and invariably choose similar seating arrangements in each semester, even if we've changed rooms.

There's probably a deep psychological reason why people choose the seats they do. Perhaps the shy ones, or others who sit in the very back, prefer to go unnoticed, while the more outgoing gravitate to the front, and those who want to blend-in stick to the middle. Maybe establishing "territories" makes them feel more comfortable.

Whatever the reason, in the long run all these pre-chosen decisions become time and confusion savers.

Only rarely—and with good reason—does a student make a change, such as when one of my gals chose another place after the man behind her repeatedly clicked his pen. Even then she felt the need to explain: "I got tired of the noise—click-click, in, out, over and over." Still, she had to be careful that she didn't usurp a location already chosen by somebody else.

One last, useful habit that just occurred to me: the minute I finish editing my student manuscripts, I put them in my briefcase—which means it's impossible to arrive in class without the homework I worked on over the week. In 35 years of teaching novel-writing, I've never arrived without my student manuscripts.

Now, having composed this section, I must choose

to make a habit out of the one area that still drives me nuts—where to place a paper that I don't wish to carry from room to room. It's a task for logic—figuring out a smart place to lay down such a sheet so I'll always know exactly where to look.

I've read that it takes a dozen repetitions to establish a "good" habit, but it also helps to reward yourself each time you do it. *Soon I'll be heading for the See's candy box.*

ALONG WITH THE CONTINUING FIGHT TO MAINTAIN our bodies, there's another important endeavor: how do we support the vital functioning of our brains?

CHAPTER FIFTEEN

Your Brain Needs Exercise, Too

IN OUR HOUSE THERE WAS ONCE A LOT OF ONGOING competition, which I freely admitted to friends, but as one of them said with a laugh, "It's rivalry just short of warfare."

For years, and for no particular reason except that we're both so competitive, Rob and I kept measuring each other, comparing what we did with what the other did, as though there was some *Otherbeing* out there keeping track. Looking back, it seems pretty silly that we debated such frivolous topics as, Who saves the most gas when he drives, Who spends the fewest minutes looking for misplaced papers, Who has the better memory.

Privately, I conceded that Rob won on memory. Except when he didn't. For a man who manages to outscore half the contestants on *Jeopardy*, it was amazing how little he remembered of my various golden words ... spoken aloud in the hope they wouldn't vanish forever.

But they vanished anyway. "Marital deafness," he said, though my friends agreed it was likely Bad Memory. Or maybe a male thing, a testosterone-driven ability to tune in or tune out. I asked Rob about this, but he didn't seem to hear me.

Still, if she was young and gorgeous, I noticed, he definitely remembered her name and most of what she said.

So, TODAY, I'VE JUST COME UP TO MY OFFICE TO GET something. But now I can't remember what on earth I came up for. The letter I just wrote? My class attendance record? Something I left on the floor?

Bugger it, I'm not going to remember, and there's lots of stuff on the floor, but not *THAT*—whatever it was.

Anyway, I'm here now, so I might as well sit down and write. The item I needed will come rushing back to my brain fairly soon; the next time I go downstairs it'll strike me, splat, as though it had been there all along.

And that's how our brains function after they've been serving us well for 80-plus years. They still work. But they're like computers with too many open files.

They're slow.

Lucky for the world, I don't work for the CIA. And you probably don't either. I'm not an airline pilot, or a doctor like our son, so it doubtless doesn't matter to anyone but me whether I remember the exact altitude of Denver, or how many bones are in the human wrist.

In the meantime, a stuttering memory is merely a nuisance. I'm tired of hearing our kids say, before

I've had a chance to ponder, "I didn't expect you to remember, Mom," or a friend grinning as she says, "I know perfectly well where I met you—but I'm having a Senior Moment."

In fact, most of us would rather we never again hear the words Senior Moment, but it is better than, "Don't I know you from somewhere?"

THERE IS A LOT OF INFORMATION AVAILABLE regarding memory loss and, while there is no magic pill (yet), most sources agree on some of the basics: Stay physically active, get enough sleep and eat a healthy, well-balanced diet. What is good for the body is also good for the brain. Some medications cause memory problems, so it is advised to regularly review your medicines with your doctor.

Socializing and learning new things (like playing a musical instrument, learning a new language, mastering a new card game, dancing, or taking up a hobby), are other tips recommended in articles by the Mayo Clinic, Harvard Health and Psychology Today.

Being better organized and having less clutter in your environment also helps. Multitasking may have been easy and useful when we were young, but focusing on one thing at a time probably helps us retain new information.

ONE OF MY MEMORY ISSUES SHOULD, BY NOW, BE A matter of habit—of asking myself a simple question whenever I leave the house: *What am I forgetting?*

For me, but not Rob, this happens all the time. I arrive at my daughter's home having left behind that elusive something I was supposed to bring.

It's easy to find excuses: a) I was running late b) I did remember one of the things c) a last-minute phone call interrupted me d) I didn't "set out" the item like I was supposed to. Bottom line: I simply forgot.

I now freely admit it—most of the time Rob doesn't have this problem. He always, or *nearly always* remembers stuff like this. But then, he's smarter than I am ... which I can acknowledge, now in my 80s, without having it hurt my ego; I've got attributes he doesn't have. Like an abundance of patience.

From the moment I met him, it was clear that Rob was an unusually smart guy ... for me, his greatest asset. Besides that, he was willing to talk. And he cared about issues I cared about.

And that brain of his—it's always been kind of won-drous hearing him supply answers to *Jeopardy!* about matters he has no business knowing. Yet one of us in the room (the patient one), is no longer bothered by an inability to come up with the name for an obscure mountain in an equally obscure country. When Rob gets it, I'm amazed, but no longer jealous.

Yet even Rob, at age 92, is mildly concerned about losing his memory. To this end, and mostly in bed, he often assigns himself memory tasks: What was the name of that neighbor who moved away 20 years ago? He works at it until he gets it. For both of us, it's an Aha! moment.

I, too, am concerned about my erratic memory— still occasional, but which usually involves something easy, like an oft-used noun. One day a friend and I couldn't, for the life of us, come up with the word "compass." I don't know about her, but it worried me down to my shoes. So, like Rob, I fight back.

When I can't remember a common word, I often let it go momentarily, while staying alert until it drifts back into memory. With that, I recite the escaped word in a variety of contexts, trying to plant it so it'll never abscond again. Or sometimes I prepare in advance for a thought I wish to impart to someone else, reciting to myself some noun which might cause me to hesitate.

Now, in this decade, Rob and I are both finding that our brains need extra stimulation, just like the rest of our bodies. To that end we both still do crossword puzzles (Rob on a daily basis). Similarly, I push my brain with numerous writing jobs—a blog when one occurs to me, or drafting pages for a current book. From the *Reader's Digest* we both take vocabulary tests. Occasionally, we memorize trivia.

Testing, always testing.

As a matter of fact, Rob almost always compiles a quiz for whenever we have a party.

WHEN MEMORY ALONE DOESN'T WORK, THE TWO OF us resort to tricks, like putting a likely-to-be-forgotten item in the middle of the family-room floor, or into the car itself. Just the act of doing this somehow reinforces our memory.

A last observation on memory—a name or thought that's associated with a strong emotion, like embarrassment, love, fear, or hate, gets irrevocably fixed in your mind. It becomes easy to remember the name of a politician you abhor—but the ones you like, not so much.

Meanwhile, around the house we find ourselves playing Taboo—when one of us can't think of a word, we talk around it until the other supplies the missing noun.

For both of us, now, our mutual cooperation on brain lapses is a lot like the way we've learned to help each other when driving the car.

For Rob and me, memory assists have become a Team Sport.

What follows are several thoughts from fellow writers: One said, "When I need to remember to take something out of the house, I fasten it to my purse with an alligator clip."

Another says, "I put stuff that goes out right in front of my door."

A third writer describes himself in his workplace, walking through the halls and inexplicably carrying a huge pile of books. Baffled, he walked into one of his fellow worker's offices. "Can you explain these? I wasn't holding them when I left."

AND HERE WE GET TO A TOPIC WHICH IS BOTH CON-cerning and embarrassing.

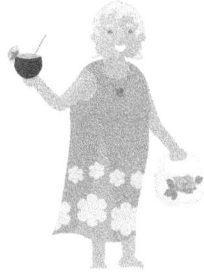

Keeping Your Southern Exposure Under Control

"Gotta hurry, rob ... gotta hurry ... hurry ... hurry. Get the door open."

After which I fly out of the car and into the house, leaving behind Rob, who's been my roommate for so many years that he knows exactly where I'm headed. The bathroom, of course.

Naturally this knowledge is private, not something either of us shares with anyone else. Yet it's one of the inevitable, call that *inevitably-unappealing* aspects of reaching your 80s.

Way back in my 40s, when I was jogging, skiing, bicycling and playing tennis, I still couldn't jump on a trampoline … not without risking a trickle of embarrassment. For most women who've had children, that one limitation begins early.

The truth is that aging involves a loss of muscle tone throughout your body: Your leg muscles, the quadriceps being one such set, are less apt to support you. The muscles in your arms (biceps), resist hoisting anything heavy and your traitorous stomach muscles (rectus abdominus), allow a new and unattractive sag of your belly. And that brings us down to the southern region and your bladder muscle (sphincter), which can also capriciously fail to protect you as it's supposed to.

With most it's possible to fight back and you don't need a gym membership or personal trainer to do it, meaning quite a few tricks can be incorporated into your everyday activities. For example, to keep the biceps toned, I deliberately lift heavy things with

one arm—a half gallon of milk, a full teakettle. Leg
and belly muscles are strengthened with leg lifts and
scissors, or stationary bicycling.

YET THE BLADDER MUSCLES THAT INSPIRE THIS
chapter are not easily controlled. In bed at night I do
Kegel exercises on a count to fifty, trying to counteract muscle weakness that comes in part from having
had too many babies.

Nurse Lauren has described "pelvic platform exercises" (as she called them), that have proven helpful
for women in this age range.

In the meantime I'm involved in an ongoing war
with that Southern part of me, determined not to be
defeated.

At all ages, life has its embarrassing moments, but
this is one we can and fervently hope to hide from the
world. However, as usual, certain tricks are involved.

First: most of us, sooner or later, are in need of
reinforcements, besides just panties. Absorbent pro-
tection comes in a variety of levels, meaning hours

of user safety. The somewhat expensive Poise is good for twelve hours (mainly during sleep), a box labeled Always, for ten hours (daytime), and the pull-ups by Depends a reliable back-up for the others.

Indelicately, at home Rob refers to these as Pee Pads. Me, not so much. The writer in me would choose a more sophisticated approach, like Wonderpads, Happynappies or Silver Liners.

What all of us most want to avoid is embarrassment. God forbid that any of us leaves a wet spot on a friend's couch. You can't just sit there, refusing to leave, until everything dries off.

Right behind that is the chagrin of finding such a spot in your own chair or bed.

The National Association For Continence (yes, there really is such an organization), estimates there are 33 million Americans dealing with some form of incontinence. There are different types and it's not always caused by age-related issues, so the first step is a check-up by your doctor.

In some cases, surgery or interventional therapies,

electrical stimulation (not sure what to think about that one), medical devices or medications are recommended. The least invasive-sounding treatments include bladder training, scheduled toilet trips, fluid and diet management, pelvic floor exercises and the aforementioned pads and protective garments.

AFTER A YEAR OF EXPERIMENTATION, IT'S BECOME clear that those embarrassing events are preventable, but you need a generous dose of self-awareness.

First, loss of control is most apt to occur under three conditions: the first is when you're working around the kitchen sink. The very sight and sounds of water seems to play havoc with a system you didn't know was listening. *Oh, boy,* I once thought to myself, *I turn on the tap and suddenly I've got to go.*

Yet even then I could recall the many recent occasions where I'd spent hours away from home without once thinking about the bathroom.

This reaction to the sound of water is a normal, conditioned response emanating from years of association: Urination *sounds* like running water and is also usually linked to the *sound* of a toilet flushing followed by hand washing. Many parents have used that sound to help potty-train their toddlers. Some research has even shown it is successful in helping adults in the treatment of shy bladder syndrome.

The second situation comes as the aftermath of a long sit. The latter can catch you entirely by surprise: you stand up, and ... whoops! a serious leak. If you've had a longish sit in the car, you realize you'll never make it safely into the house.

The third, not surprising at all, is when the call of nature wakes you in the middle of the night.

All three have solutions—and here the bathroom becomes your friend. In most houses there's a utility bath somewhere near the kitchen. If, like me, your greatest consumption of liquids is in the morning, you're prepared, physically and mentally, for frequent bathroom runs.

The second situation is generally a surprise—but now preventable with prophylactic potty trips.

Among these are: before going upstairs for long sits at the computer; before leaving your house to go anywhere; before leaving somebody else's house or the restaurant to come home.

In the absence of such foresight, there's another trick: before you rise from chair or car seat, do a series of kegel exercises; often they'll calm down your bladder and allow you to safely reach the bathroom.

Nothing is worse than that sense of impending disaster as you arrive home. Whatever else you try doesn't work. You'll soon have to change everything, from outside to in. Most annoying, the shoes must come off before all the rest.

The third and most common overflow situation occurs in the middle of the night. Yet that's the most easily handled. First, savvy seniors tend to avoid much liquid late in the day. Next, with an extra-absorbent Poise pad, followed by a Depends pull-up, you're in safe territory from bedtime to get-up.

YOUR GYNOCOLOGIST HAS A NUMBER OF BLADDER

and urethra surgeries for bladder prolapse and/or stress incontinence. I won't attempt to describe or evaluate them here. Fortunately, most elderly women can avoid urologic surgery with adequate changes in lifestyle.

WHILE THIS ISSUE MAY BE THE MOST EMBARRASSING part of being 80, it needn't impact your life in a mortifying way or prevent you from continuing to live as an active, productive citizen. The solutions are simple and twofold: buying the most useful of the various products on the market, and taking more potty breaks than you ever thought you'd need.

Once the necessary adjustments are made, you may not sign up for a trampoline contest or trip the light fantastic, but you can lead a reasonably normal life as a Golden Oldie.

UNTIL TWO CARELESS EVENTS DISRUPTED MY LIFE, I wouldn't have thought it necessary to discuss a problem as elementary as cuts and scratches.

CHAPTER SEVENTEEN

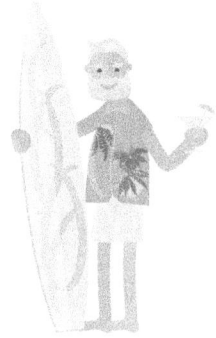

It's Only A Flesh Wound

FOR MOST OF US, OCCASIONAL SCRAPES AND scratches have long been a routine part of life. In fact, I once owned a Lincoln Town Car that, like an ill-tempered cat, regularly attacked me. The driver's side door was poorly designed, meaning it curved inward like a scimitar, so that just exiting the vehicle meant you were apt to suffer an enormous gash in your leg.

In those days even a severe scrape became an annoyance that lasted only a couple of weeks, because things like that healed so quickly. However, I soon tired of finding myself with blood seeping through my slacks, and I returned the car to the dealer ... before it ripped my leg off.

Not long after, I happened to be talking to a good friend, and found she, too, returned her Town Car—and for the same reason. We were then both in our late 60s, and indignant that some impervious, out-of-touch, style-oriented engineer had designed such a patently dangerous driver's-side door. We wondered how many other owner-legs had suffered similar wounds.

Today, in my 80s, a scrape like that would be both serious and perhaps even dangerous.

It's a fact that healing is slower in later years than it was in the first half of our lives. We seniors do heal, and thank heavens for that, but like everything else we experience, the process is sluggish.

As we move at a more deliberative pace, so does our inflammatory response, which allows blood vessels to expand and send nutrients and white blood cells (the soldiers of our body),to a wound. If those warriors can't get to a wound to fight bacteria and infection, we are in trouble. Reduced skin elasticity also can affect how fast you heal. According to the U.S. National Library of Medicine, having thin skin can make wound healing four times slower.

Diabetes is another culprit. A 2015 CDC report indicates that more than 100 million American adults are living with diabetes or prediabetes conditions. Elevated blood sugar levels can significantly hamper wound healing.

As a further issue, legs traditionally heal slower than other parts of the body. As our son, Chris, explained, the blood supply to one's legs is not as abundant or as fast-acting as in arms and elsewhere. Even my recent orthopedist, much younger than I am, had minor leg surgery that took a full four weeks to heal.

WITH THAT, I'LL SHARE TWO EVENTS THAT SEEMED minor at the time, but ended up scaring me because the injuries obviously weren't healing. The first happened in the kitchen, where the dishwasher was open, with the door down and protruding into the room. In my usual haste to unload it, I circled the open door, but came too close with my bare right leg. To my horror, the sharp-edged corner peeled back about an inch and a half of skin. (Did I mention that age makes our skin increasingly friable, meaning thin, delicate, and easily torn?)

The pain wasn't significant, but the look of it was. I staggered over to Rob, who was horrified. He applied an antibiotic salve and a bandage.

The days went by and our applications of salve continued, but it soon became apparent that nothing was helping. Finally, when the wound began bubbling, I showed it to Chris. "You need an antibiotic," he said, "and you need an immediate visit with your G.P." It was then a late-Friday afternoon, and luckily I caught my family doctor just before she left the office.

She took one look and said, in effect, "This is beyond me, you need to see my husband." (An orthopedic surgeon.) She got me in immediately, and he cleaned the wound and prescribed many weeks of two different antibiotics. For a while, I seemed to be swallowing pills nonstop.

Then nurse Lauren got involved, from up in Tahoe, and soon I was sending her frequent pictures of the lesion. Reports on the leg became something of a family affair. Lauren advised me to elevate it, which you can only do by lying down. Those were the weeks when Rob and Tracy brought in nonstop meals, and I managed to read two whole books.

Eventually I was rewarded with long-distance cheering, as the gash began healing, and eventually scabbed over nicely. Though now completely healed, the wound left behind a memento—a bright red spot on my lower leg.

"That area will always be sensitive," Lauren said, "you need to rub it with lotion."

"Okay," I said, and since then that spot has been babied and rewarded with regular, sweet-smelling body creams.

IRONICALLY, MONTHS LATER, A MINOR SCRAPE ON another part of that same leg produced a second small injury that also failed to heal. But this time the slight abrasion required only a ten-day course of a single antibiotic. Eventually it, too, gave up its mean-spirited grip on my body and finally healed.

My purpose for relating all this is to demonstrate that even innocuous leg wounds can be dangerous in our eighties. As we've probably all done until now, we need to pay attention to what our bodies are telling us.

But more important still, is being alert for objects in our environment that stick out or have sharp edges which are liable to bump, scratch, or scrape us. Friable skin isn't apparent to anyone except those of us who live inside it. Like other parts of us, our skin needs to be jealously protected.

The truth is, to avoid injury of every sort means being on constant patrol for those seemingly inno-cent things all around that can rear up unexpectedly, like a cobra, and attack without warning.

Meanwhile, I wonder how long it took Lincoln to re-design the saber door on that malevolent model.

SINCE FEW OF US STILL ASPIRE TO BE MOVIE STARS, it's easy to take a casual, *what the hell* attitude about how we look. Yet looking our best is more than its own reward.

CHAPTER EIGHTEEN

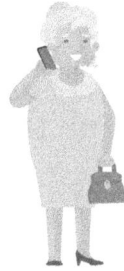

Your Face Is Your Billboard

RECENTLY A MAN IN THE NEWS MADE THE COMMENT, "If I'd known I was going to be on a Wanted poster, I'd have tried to look better."

As a matter of fact, a few celebrities, like Dolly Parton, Jane Fonda, and Leslie Stahl, who were smart enough to grasp they couldn't retain their youthful looks forever, nevertheless took steps to remain as attractive as possible—with the result that they're still taken seriously as performers. Leslie Stahl has lately toned down her famous, electric red lipstick.

Until recently, when you saw her on *Sixty Minutes*, she was all lips.

And Dolly Parton has joked, "It costs a lot of money to look this cheap."

Way back when, I remember thinking, *When I hit 70* (as the century changes), *I won't care about anything—how I look or what's going on around me.*

How wrong I was! At 70, and now in my 80s, I've discovered that I still care intensely about everything—my appearance, and what is happening in the larger world.

So yes, among my critics are Rob and the bathroom mirror. Both are programmed to tell the truth. I still buy new clothes (now only occasionally), and pay lots of attention to my hair. I regularly renew my lipstick, and I still care which shoes I'm wearing ... meaning before a social event the tennies get shucked in favor of pumps.

Of course all my footwear is now flat ... reinforced by son, Chris, drawing on numerous medical lectures, often titled, "High-heeled shoes: the work of the devil." When asked to elaborate, he said, "Your foot's not made to walk on your tippy-toes. In fact, we see more surgeries due to faulty shoes than any other one cause."

Recently, a friend mailed me a card which I loved and showed to everyone. The entire message was on the front: "Slap on a little lipstick … you'll be fine." Inside, her handwritten note told us, "That's what my mother always used to say."

My Mom seldom gave me advice, so the lipstick issue was mine to figure out. That card was made for me. All my life I've tried not to go anywhere without *slapping on* a streak of *Frosted Apricot*. Having years ago discovered the one brand and the one color that suits me—and for which I sometimes get compliments—it's still a regular part of getting dressed. As my son said when he chose his wife at age 16: "Mom, when you find what you're looking for, why go on shopping?"

Well, the same can be said for lipstick.

Here another bias emerges. To offset the drab

aura created by dark browns and blacks, but mainly because I like them, I've always worn lively hues— bright pinks, reds, aquas, electric blues, sometimes vivid yellows. Namely, the colors worn by children.

You notice that kids seldom wear black.

Nor do I.

Even in college I never owned that mandatory "little black dress." Since to me they all appeared to be the same dress, they fell into the category of a uniform. *How can anyone love black*, I wondered, *it's so boring.*

Well, there go all my readers from New York City.

WITH MY WEIGHT NOW BACK TO COLLEGE DAYS, (thanks to those two meals a day), I've discovered that all the items in my too-many-clothes wardrobe still fit. And no longer are dress-up outfits saved for that rare elegant occasion. They get worn, willy-nilly, with the question, *What am I saving this FOR?*

And so it goes with people in our age group—some put in extra effort to look their best, while a few seem not to care. In fact, it's always startling to see older women on television with hair that makes no effort to enhance their faces, or lips that remain dull and colorless.

And here a last note about my mother-in-law, Ruth. Until the end, even in the hospital, she wore a wig. But the odd thing about the wig was that it wasn't a youthful color; instead, the hair was a nice shade of gray. Underneath, her own hair was still black. She explained with a touch of scorn, "Black hair is all wrong for a woman my age."

AT ALL AGES, BUT ESPECIALLY NOW, REMAINING reasonably attractive requires at least four elements: a) good genes, b) lots of sleep, c) a healthy diet, and d) exercise (even exercise of the face.)

The good news is remarkably good; we do have some control over at least three of these elements. Genetics are pre-determined, but clearly the rest are not. As described in the chapters on sleep and food, we can take steps to enhance our health and our lives—which also include appearance. As to exercise, however much it promotes general health, an additional plus is better looks.

Specific to facial attractiveness are the two routines covered in the book, "Be a Loser." A) An antidote to sagging cheeks requires, for a count of ten, simultaneously sucking in your stomach and sticking out your tongue—extending it as far as possible toward your chin— and B) Again sucking in your stomach while puckering up your lips into a fish mouth and holding them for a count of ten. Each should be done daily, with five repetitions per maneuver. Taken together, both help maintain muscle tone in our faces.

A reminder: I suggest you refrain from doing this in public, as I once did—the time my hairdresser asked if she should call an ambulance.

I, for one, have never used facial makeup; from my grandmother I was lucky enough to inherit fairly good skin. I wash my face daily with any old soap, and afterwards apply the inexpensive lubricant, *Aquaphor*. To my surprise, when I asked my dermatologist if they knew about that product, she said, "Oh, *Aquaphor!* We love it!"

As an alternative to facial exercise, women with resources are apt to choose face lifts, with varying results from great to awful. A friend recently reported that she'd been to a literary luncheon where almost everyone at her table had clearly undergone such a procedure. "All those tight faces," she said. "As a group, they made it so obvious."

"But did they look good?" I asked, envisioning a table full of women wearing the same alert, slightly surprised expressions.

"Not really. They all looked post-surgical." She shrugged. "None of them made me want to have one."

Yet I know a very special woman, a celebrity whom I'll call Jane, whose face lift was so enhancing, she appeared years and years younger than her true age, while offering no sign she'd had anything done. When she told me about it, she said, "My doctor has asked me to stop recommending him to my friends ..." She laughed. "He can no longer deal with so many women who want his services."

I've observed other women, including my aunt, whose post-surgical face was so tight and shiny she appeared to have been the victim of a fire. Sadly, with most women I've known (but not Jane), the beneficial effects seem to wear off within a few years, leaving them more wrinkled than ever.

Yet judging by the excellent appearances of so many aging Hollywood stars, plastic surgery is a fine art—and the best practitioners seem to have set up shop in Hollywood.

WRINKLES AND SAGGING JOWLS AREN'T THE ONLY skin tribulations we seniors have to deal with. Dry, itchy skin, age spots, skin tags and, even more serious, skin cancer, are all concerns that become more prevalent with each passing year. As mentioned earlier, aging skin becomes thinner, loses fat and no longer looks soft and plump. (If only our fat would lose fat so efficiently.)

The National Institute on Aging recommends

drinking more fluids and limiting sun exposure, as well as applying lotion daily and using a humidifier if your environment is dry.

However, using too much soap, antiperspirant or perfume can exacerbate dry skin issues, as can soaking in very hot baths.

Some medicines and health problems—like diabetes or kidney disease–also can cause dry skin, so if you experience a sudden change, mention it to your doctor.

Skin tags are small growths that become common as we age, especially on the eyelids, neck and body folds, such as the armpits, chest and groin areas. Like age spots, which are the result of sun damage, skin tags are generally harmless, and if they bother you, can easily be removed by a dermatologist.

Skin cancer, however, is a much more serious issue. Years of unprotected sun exposure in our youth can come back to haunt us in our later years. The most common types are basal cell carcinoma and squamous cell carcinoma, which grow slowly and are rarely life-threatening.

The third and most dangerous type of skin cancer is melanoma, which can spread to other organs and be deadly. So, as you are smearing the lotion on your "mature" skin, check for any new growths, sores that don't heal, and bleeding or itchy moles.

Your dermatologist will know which lesions to leave alone, which to zap, and which need further doctoring.

UNFAIRLY, WHEN IT COMES TO LOOKS, THE GENERAL public is subconsciously biased; the better we look, the better we tend to be treated. Too often, seniors are dismissed as being merely *old*, and probably not worth engaging in conversation. How wrong that can be!

BACK IN OUR THIRTIES AND FORTIES, WHEN ROB AND I were still considered young, we often found ourselves out-aged at certain events, such as at the *World Affairs Council*. I remember groaning inwardly at the prospect of being seated at a table comprised mostly of folks who seemed *ancient.* Both Rob and I were anticipating tedious, lackluster table conversations. But we were soon riveted by the interesting dialogues swirling around us, the accumulated wisdom and the seniors' compelling life experiences. Even as they spoke, the years dropped away and they appeared younger and more vibrant. Invariably we came away commenting to each other, "What a surprise!" "I can't believe it—those couples were downright fascinating!"

Yet even then, like others our age, we had to get past first impressions.

THAT SAID, IT'S TIME TO DISCUSS ANOTHER COMPEL-ling issue that afflicts too many oldsters. How do we deal with the ever-present threat of isolation?

CHAPTER NINETEEN

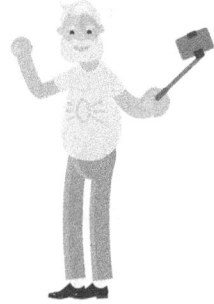

One Is A Lonely Number

HENRY THOREAU MAY HAVE RELISHED SOLITUDE ON Walden Pond, but nobody would recommend it for an octogenarian. A lot of peace and quiet may be good for a composer or poet, but it can lead to depression for a solitary senior if it comes in large doses.

A study by the University of California San Francisco found that loneliness increases the likelihood of death by 26 percent and that Medicare patients who live alone spend about $130 more a month on healthcare needs. Researchers also found that seniors who feel isolated have a 64 percent greater chance of developing clinical dementia.

Even elderly couples are wise to maintain a fair degree of socializing after retirement and after their families have disappeared over the horizon, some to other states.

This is especially hard for a new widow, because friends and acquaintances tend to socialize in pairs. Many a widow has discovered to her dismay that she has seemingly lost contact with some of her couple friends ... without the friends realizing their abandonment. Yet it's hard to blame the paired-off friends who fail to invite her along, because she's always an odd number.

The same can't be said for new widowers, who are invariably in short supply. Suddenly they find themselves on the casserole circuit, regularly treated to delicious food by the stereotypical brave or love-starved widows.

There are no hard statistics on the ratio of widows

and widowers who remarry, but the U.S. Census Bureau estimates that in the over-age-60 category, ten times as many men remarry as do women, though there are considerably fewer men in that age group.

Loneliness, combined with some of the issues we've already discussed—hearing and vision loss, the fear of falling and the inability to drive—can leave a senior, especially a woman, feeling like she is a prisoner in her own home.

WHERE ONCE ROB AND I CONSIDERED IT ANATHEMA to find ourselves with nothing to do on a Saturday night, we now mind far less than we once did. In fact, I, for one, have so many regularly-scheduled "away" evenings, that it's often a treat just to stay home watching television with Rob.

Among my pre-set nights are Mondays with a writing-critique group and Wednesdays teaching a class in Novel and Memoir writing. Added to those are daytime events, such as the writing workshop I teach at a friend's home, plus regular luncheons with women friends.

And these are not all. Rob and I are lucky enough that two of our children live nearby, where we're frequently invited to dinner. The two of us now have the same feelings of delight at going to our children's houses that we once experienced attending a lively couples' event at our church.

With Rob waiting for me at home after my several "away" events, those old, occasional feelings of being left out are gone.

Still, it's no stretch to imagine that loneliness is a regular feature for lots of people in their 80s. From that, depression is likely to follow.

For these souls, it appears the best remedy is trying to be pro-active, to seek out excuses for social interaction. Many urban communities, such as ours, sponsor a Senior Center, replete with nearly-free luncheons and a variety of special classes ... groups that gather for crafts, writing, exercise, book clubs, swimming, painting, or quilting. Here they'll find other seniors with similar interests and the potential of becoming friends.

Our local Presbyterian Church (and other churches), sponsor programs designed specifically for folks in their 70s and 80s. Among them would be book clubs and group excursions to well-recognized entertainment or cultural centers, such as sports events, The Hollywood Bowl, or Laguna Beach's Festival of The Arts.

Another outlet would be volunteering. Seniors are generally welcomed when they volunteer to tutor book-needy children in our crowded local schools. It takes nothing more than imagination and patience to work one-on-one with a child who's slipping behind in reading or math.

Other such pursuits might be helping to parcel out groceries in food banks, or playing waiter as they serve food to the homeless. Our local thrift stores depend on the help they get from seniors who are volunteers.

Whatever a senior did before as a parent or wage-earner would probably be useful in the world of volunteers. An ex-musician, for instance, could help teach elementary children the rudiments of playing a musical instrument. As a talented senior digs deeper into his once-active life, he will surely unearth skills that would be useful to pass on to others.

Support groups for the arts, or certain diseases, are eager to accept volunteers of whatever age.

Last but not least, if an octogenerian's home features a spare bedroom, it's always possible, with important attention to screening, to bring in a renter who will provide a modicum of company. This would be feasible only if there's a nearby relative or friend who could make regular visits to check on the arrangement.

Rob and I have been rewarded by travel—especially when we've taken grandchildren on vacation trips—always stimulating and great fun, if it's within your budget.

FOR SENIORS WHO LIVE IN FACILITIES DEDICATED TO older age groups, it's already clear that anyone who might otherwise be lonely can participate in a great variety of activities. One glance at their posted schedule says it all: movie nights; designated trips to a mall; excursions to live theatre; special bingo nights; celebratory parties; in-house dances with a disk jockey or band; an hour dedicated to an entertainer or speaker.

I can vouch for the acceptability of lectures from the outside. Over the years I've spoken about my books and writing in general at more than half a dozen senior centers—and, on numerous occasions, to a few communities, such as Leisure World.

There are even stories of seniors finding late-in-life romance after moving into one of these facilities. A friend recently recounted the tale of two elderly women getting into a hair-pulling, walker-shoving tussle when they discovered they were "dating" the same elderly gentleman, who had apparently been attending different meal seatings so he could keep the ladies apart.

THERE'S AN OLD SAYING THAT KEEPS COMING BACK to me: *You can choose whether to be happy.*

I would hasten to add, "Under normal circum-stances." By this, I mean happiness would be difficult or impossible for plenty of people … the homeless, perhaps, or someone living in constant pain. Or after the loss of someone you hold dear. Nobody would be foolish enough to claim that happiness is available to everyone under all conditions.

Yet every day, in newspapers or on television, we find examples of individuals who choose joy when they'd be justified to wallow in misery.

I'm thinking about the always-dramatic television program, *On The Road—With Steve Hartman*. One of his episodes describes a tall, thin and stooped senior citizen who'd lost his wife and saw no reason to go on living. Yet one day as he hobbled about the grocery store, a little girl, about four, reached out to him from her market basket seat and said, "Hey, old man, it's my birthday!"

The man looked up, at first startled, but then he smiled and the girl's mother smiled too. When the child continued to beckon him over, he could tell it was okay to engage the little girl. He came closer, and the child babbled on, as though she'd known him forever. Eventually, he walked the pair to their car.

From there a close friendship developed between the man and his new little pal. The "old man" was invited to the girl's house for visits, and soon they were nearly inseparable. It's as though the fellow had acquired a lively new granddaughter, and she, in turn, had found a much-needed friend.

All of a sudden he had something to look forward to. Happiness returned to the man's life. But he *chose* to let his new, unexpected friendship brighten his days. Clearly, just under the surface, joy was waiting to be re-ignited.

Among Steve Hartman's many touching shows, this remains one of our favorites … an example of how loneliness can sometimes be dispelled in the most surprising of encounters … and often when it's least expected.

WHAT FOLLOWS NEXT ARE A FEW TIDBITS ABOUT OUR current lives … about facing down tragedy and finding joy in our ongoing days.

CHAPTER TWENTY

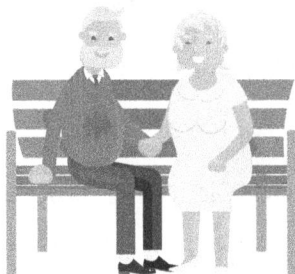

It's Attitude That Keeps us Going

NOBODY GETS TO AGE EIGHTY WITHOUT EXPERIENC-
ing one or more tragedies. For starters, by then you've
lost both parents. Even when death is expected, it
comes as a shock.

Worse, most of us have suffered heartbreaks beyond
the deaths of our parents—events that reached down
and threatened to destroy us and, for a time, tore at
our very souls.

I once supposed our daughter—beautiful, smart,
vivacious, with endless friends—might be one person

who was destined to "have it all." That is, until she lost her first husband to melanoma, then later a second partner to a brain tumor.

As for Rob and me, we've suffered the deaths of two sons, taken from us at ages 20 and 27, both in hang gliding accidents.

How do you deal with such tragedies? How do you come out of such grief, months later, still able to smile—and yes, even laugh?

In our neighborhood, years ago, we were given an example of tragedy that overtook a family and never released the parents from its clutches. In a sad, almost inevitable way, the two chose to let unending grief become the mantra that set the tone for the rest of their lives.

Here were the parents of four children, living happily in a nice home, with the father a successful doctor. One day the unthinkable happened: a son was killed on the freeway, the victim of a runaway truck. Their close friends reacted with expected sympathy and ongoing support.

Time passed and life went on around them, yet for some reason the parents never recovered from their loss. Within their home they created a shrine to the missing son, with a candle that was never allowed to go out. Ultimately, the three surviving children became the victims of their parents' grief—as though their lives no longer mattered. Eventually, to save themselves, two of the boys retreated into situations that had nothing to do with their parents.

While close friends continued to offer support, it soon became clear that those parents' only concern was their never-ending tragedy … a permanent obstacle to happiness in any form.

Since both our losses preceded theirs, they once asked, "How did you get over your grief?"

I, at least, never knew what to say. In retrospect, honesty might have compelled an answer, which the two doubtless would have ignored: "We never got over it, but we did get through it. Part of the reason is, we still had other kids to love. We concentrated on *them*."

In truth, our healing was more complicated than that.

FROM THE DEATH OF OUR THIRD-BORN SON, ERIC, Rob and I learned our first hard lessons about grief and survival, truisms nobody would choose to explore in advance. I remember, for instance, that my father, offering comfort, flew out to California from Long Island, and soon after the funeral he suggested that we all go play tennis.

I was shocked. *How can I play and enjoy myself when my son has just died?* The whole idea felt blasphemous.

As I recall, neither of us expressed our reluctance, so in lieu of objecting we simply played. And for that short hour our minds became focused elsewhere, and perhaps that was when the healing began.

Rob's attitude then was both instructive and helpful. "Life goes on," he said, "and we focus on the present and future, not on the past."

At the same time, we also learned something about

sorrow itself, how it manifests with most of us. We discovered that grief comes in waves. At first, for a short period, you may feel you're back to normal, but then a wave hits and knocks you flat, right back to where you started. It's always unexpected, a shock, and for awhile this keeps happening.

Eventually, you begin to notice a change. The waves get smaller and they're not as frequent. As you return to normal living, there comes a time when you realize you haven't thought about your loss for most of a day. And slowly (different for everyone), that day becomes several in a row.

Bit by bit, ever so subtly, the pain recedes. All the while it helps if you have other loved ones to think and care about, and the sense that you're engaged with life and doing something worthwhile.

Even so, at the same time it feels unworthy and all wrong to ever stop missing your loved one. For many of us the sense of loss never fades entirely. The best we can hope for is a return to normalcy, with the person you loved in a distant, rearview mirror.

A DIFFERENT LESSON CAME TO ME WITH OUR SECOND tragedy, with the loss of our oldest son, Bobby. From the awful moment I realized he'd died, I didn't think I'd survive. *How can a mother live through the deaths of two sons?*

I honestly expected my body would give out and I'd suddenly keel over in shock. It never happened. Instead, I stumbled along in a kind of numb haze. A year later I wrote about our two sons in a memoir, *Higher Than Eagles*, and found that putting emotions on paper seems to lift the full impact off your psyche—as though the paper absorbs some of what you've been feeling. I never expected it to be cathartic, though in fact it probably was.

ALL OUR LIVES WE'VE NOTICED TWO KINDS OF 80-year-olds: those who are grumpy, silent, and no fun to be around, and a whole lot of others who manage to tell great stories, to listen attentively, and to laugh with genuine pleasure at whatever craziness comes their way.

I had a mother-in-law who was a little bit of both. At times I'd find her grumpy and fearful—yet I was usually able to entertain her with my latest, mostly-humorous story of a non-tragic foul-up. I found myself saving those tidbits to relay to Ruth on our regular visits. Even in her last few days, Ruth herself was able to summon a few quips to entertain three of her great-grandchildren. Consequently, Ruth had more visitors than the usual 94-year-old.

Now, suddenly, here I am … today's version of Ruth. Still, I'm a few years younger and not in physical peril.

WE'VE SEEN COUNTLESS EXAMPLES OF HAPPINESS radiating from seniors who make a decision to help others. As noted in the prior chapter, some serve food at homeless shelters or retirement communities. Others collect useful items to give away, or join libraries where they read stories to children.

Friends of mine are quilters, making colorful bed covers for the poor. A few seniors volunteer to drive non-driving oldsters to doctor's appointments.

Nearly all those who choose to help others do so, at least in part, because the happiness they create bounces back to *them*. A smile of thanks or an expression of gratitude from someone you've served is like running it through a magnifying mirror ... it rebounds in the giver's direction, but also seems to return multiplied.

FOR SOME OF US, PLEASURE DERIVES WHEN WE KEEP working—doing whatever it is we've done most of our lives. Thus, I continue to teach novel-writing, and on the side I also write books. Never mind that I've already published some 19 volumes. I couldn't bear to wake up each morning with no goal in mind, with *nothing special to do.*

Because I'm constantly tuned to national news, opinions and responses pour into my psyche. Perhaps oftener than I should, I can't resist speaking out to the larger world, usually in the form of a blog. The excitement comes when, over the course of a week, I discover that more than a hundred people, mostly strangers, have chosen to read what I posted. A few even respond.

Rob is also a writer. He turns out frequent insightful, philosophical, and political essays, which he sends to family and enthusiastic friends. Over the last few years he's published them in three different volumes. Like me, he wants the world to know what he's thinking, though he's less apt than I am to lecture gratuitously to anyone who'll listen.

For each of us, it's fulfilling to constantly view the world through a writer's eye.

SAVING THE BEST FOR LAST, HAPPINESS POURS INTO us "oldies" from our family—and almost equally from our friends. By age 80, not many of us have the energy to throw large parties at home … or even small ones with one to three other couples. Playing host and hostess can be exhausting, with all the house-straightening, the cooking, the setting of tables, the flowers, the serving of food, the cleaning-up afterwards.

Yet most of us can afford to play host at a restaurant,

or, alternatively, meet friends somewhere with an unspoken agreement that each party pays his own way.

The world's saddest 80-year-olds must be those who've chosen, at earlier ages, to pick fights with their once-best-friends or family members ... and thus to arrive in their 80s with no one they're close to.

Like it or not, nourishing friendships at any age requires a modicum of effort. Overlooking minor disagreements, or even the occasional perceived slight requires forbearance, and means you don't take every social bump as the final word in a relationship.

With that said, Rob and I find our lives still rich, still full of laughter from our very large family. We now have 10 grandchildren and 14 great grandchildren. Plus we are lucky enough to feel warm connections to an assortment of friends.

IF THE ABOVE SOUNDS A BIT CORNY, FOR ROB AND me, our final thoughts on being in our late 80s (in Rob's case, 92), is that you do the best you can to maintain your physical body. But you work just as hard at seeing the positives that are still part of your daily existence.

About the Author

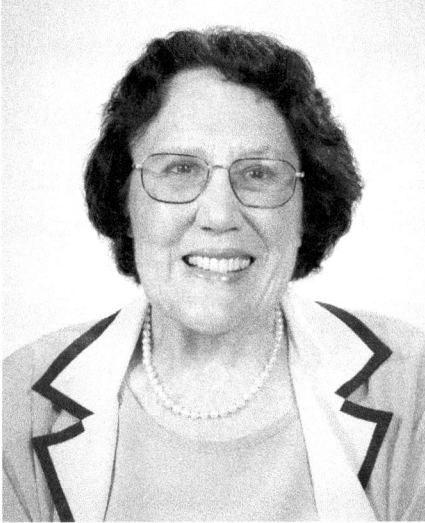

MARALYS WILLS HAS LIVED THREE DISTINCT LIVES: author of 19 published books, teacher of college students, and mother of six children—five boys and a girl.

Educated at Stanford and UCLA, she is married to a retired trial attorney. She currently teaches novel writing on the college level, and in 2000 was named Teacher of the Year.

Her most challenging project, a poignant memoir titled *Higher Than Eagles,* became her biggest triumph, garnering excellent reviews and five movie options.

Wills considers public speaking the dessert for all the hard work of writing, and relishes every moment spent with a receptive audience. She welcomes readers' input.

Contact her: maralys@cox.net or www.maralys.com

Word of mouth is crucial for any author to succeed. If you enjoyed this book, please consider leaving a review on Amazon, even if it's only a line or two; it will make all the difference and is very much appreciated.

www.ingramcontent.com/pod-product-compliance
Lightning Source LLC
Chambersburg PA
CBHW071012280326
41934CB00025B/3042